INSECURITY
DETOX

A Breakout Plan to Rejuvenate Your Body, Mind, and Spirit

Trish Blackwell

Foreword by Todd Durkin, MA, CSCS, Author of *The IMPACT Body Plan*
and Trainer to NFL, NBA, MLB & Olympic Champion Athletes

HOWARD BOOKS
An Imprint of Simon & Schuster, Inc.
New York   Nashville   London   Toronto   Sydney   New Delhi

Howard Books
An Imprint of Simon & Schuster, Inc.
1230 Avenue of the Americas
New York, NY 10020

First Howard Books trade paperback edition April 2016

HOWARD and colophon are trademarks of Simon & Schuster, Inc.

Published in association with William K. Jensen Literary Agency, 119 Bampton Court, Eugene, OR 97404.

For information about special discounts for bulk purchases, please contact Simon & Schuster Special Sales at 1-866-506-1949 or business@simonandschuster.com

The Simon & Schuster Speakers Bureau can bring authors to your live event. For more information or to book an event contact the Simon & Schuster Speakers Bureau at 1-866-248-3049 or visit our website at www.simonspeakers.com.

Interior design by Davina Mock-Maniscalco

Manufactured in the United States of America

10   9   8   7   6   5   4   3   2   1

Library of Congress Control Number: 2015038215

ISBN 978-1-5011-2130-2
ISBN 978-1-5011-2133-3 (ebook)

For Ellie, may your heart be filled with God's love and confidence and may it spill out onto others with infectious joy. I love you completely.

CONTENTS

FOREWORD   vii

INTRODUCTION   xiii

DETOX 1: Expectations   1

DETOX 2: Emotional Baggage   11

DETOX 3: Old Patterns   19

DETOX 4: Negative Self-Talk   27

DETOX 5: Trying to Be Someone Else   37

DETOX 6: Unworth   45

DETOX 7: Control   55

DETOX 8: The Ordinary   75

DETOX 9: Limited Thinking   83

DETOX 10: Untapped Potential   93

DETOX 11: Self-Doubt   99

DETOX 12: Busyness   109

DETOX 13: The Destination   117

DETOX 14: Incompleteness 125

DETOX 15: External Affirmation 133

DETOX 16: Distorted Perception 141

DETOX 17: The Mirror 151

DETOX 18: Perfectionistic Thinking 159

DETOX 19: Fear 167

DETOX 20: Negativity 177

DETOX 21: Lack of Confidence 185

DETOX 22: Small Dreams 193

DETOX 23: The Marked Path 203

DETOX 24: Negative Body Image 211

DETOX 25: Pessimistic Perspective 221

DETOX 26: A Boring Life 231

DETOX 27: Narrow Worldview 241

DETOX 28: Lack of Focus 251

DETOX 29: Past Hurts 261

DETOX 30: Lack of Routine 269

30 Detoxes Review Guide 277

Acknowledgments 287

FOREWORD

I believe all of us have a life worth telling a story about—a story that can make a profound difference in other people's lives.

Many of us have faced adversity, heartache, challenge, setback, and insecurity. Sometimes life seems too busy, too overwhelming, and downright defeating. I have always said that adversity and challenge can do one of several things to you:

1) It can create fear and insecurity that knocks you down, keeps you down, and spirals you into a deep, dark place.

2) It can propel you forward if you ultimately choose to do something positive with your life.

3) Or it can do both!

As a performance coach, trainer, author, speaker, and business owner, I have had the opportunity to work with many high-level athletes and executives. From NFL MVPs, Super Bowl champions and MVPs, MLB and NBA All-Stars, and Olympic gold medalists to the uber-successful entrepreneur who is worth billions of dollars. Literally.

All the great ones I know and have worked with have one thing in common: they have all overcome adversity. Lack of belief. Injury. Disease. Bankruptcy. Divorce. Family tragedy. Tough childhood. Failed businesses. Fear. And more.

Now I am not saying you have to experience terrible adversity to be successful in life. You don't.

But this is the bottom line: good things and bad things will come into your life. And there are some things you can control and some you can't.

But no matter what happens in your life, you can choose how you respond. One of the mantras I live by is "Get your mind right." Choose to do everything possible to live in a stratosphere that allows your body, mind, and spirit to soar.

This takes work.

It takes daily practice.

It takes solid routines.

It takes discipline and consistent effort.

It takes surrounding yourself with the right people.

It takes reading and listening to messages that manifest positivity and inspiration.

And all of this is a *choice*.

Are you ready to choose to be the best version of yourself and to live a life worth telling a story about?

Let me introduce you to my friend Trish Blackwell. She can help you.

I have known Trish for more than five years now, and I've worked with her extensively on many levels. She is a coach. A trainer. An author. A podcaster. A mom. A wife. And an extraordinary human being.

And she can help you be your *best*.

In this new book, *Insecurity Detox: A Breakout Plan to Rejuvenate Your Body, Mind, and Spirit,* Trish will inspire and empower you from the inside out. Her thirty progressive, step-by-step detoxes will boost your confidence, empower your soul, and allow you to live with the confidence and faith to be your best.

Trish is open, honest, and authentic about her Christian faith and how it plays an important role in how you live out your deepest passion and purpose in life. I love how Trish provides a daily Bible verse to reinforce each one of her detox messages and to help you get your mind right.

Does it take work to be your best? You bet it does. And it sometimes takes "divorcing your story" to cleanse your body, mind, and spirit.

Trish's book and program *will* help.

When you read Trish's book and follow her program, you will discover . . .

1) *Hope.* Hope for your future and the abundance that life offers you. Your passion will be reignited and your purpose will deepen.

2) *Confidence.* Confidence is who Trish is. She's a confidence coach who will work miracles in your body, mind, and soul. By following her plan, you *will* become more confident.

3) *Belief.* Belief that you can rid yourself of any bonds or chains that may be holding you back.

4) *Vibrancy*. Trish's suggested physical exercises will allow you to get your brain and body operating at world-class levels. Your energy will soar, and your smile will radiate positivity.

5) *Motivation*. Motivation to be a better parent. A better spouse. A better person.

6) *Inspiration*. Inspiration to be your best . . . and then some. Motivation is in the mind. Inspiration is in the heart. You will be both motivated and inspired.

7) *Gratefulness*. Gratefulness for what and Who is in your life.

8) *Love*. All of Trish's work epitomizes love. This new book and program is no different. You will feel the most powerful emotion you can experience for yourself and for others: *love*!

My friend, when I say that "Everyone has a life worth telling a story about . . . what's your story?"™, I mean it. It is true. You have a life worth telling a story about. But it's up to you to choose to do something extraordinary with your life.

And the more adversity and challenge you have faced in the past or that you are facing now, the more people you can ultimately influence and impact. But you must be willing to act and overcome. Trish's program provides a life-plan to help you do this.

Trish, from the bottom of my heart, thank you for having the courage to be you. To share so openly and genuinely. And thank you for sharing your story. It has not only made me a better person, I am confident that your story is going to motivate, inspire, and impact thousands of other people as well.

As I conclude, please remember this foundational truth, which you'll discover in Trish's story, book, and program: regardless of your background, age, race, sex, education, "hand you were dealt," and your current success or failure, you were created to be special, and greatness is your destiny.

After all, you do have a life worth telling a story about. Now is your time to get up, take action to get what you want, and create the life you desire.

Keep your faith, dream big, and always, always . . . create *impact*.

Much love.

Todd Durkin, MA, CSCS
Owner, Fitness Quest 10
Lead Training Advisor, Under Armour
Author, *The IMPACT Body Plan*
Trainer to NFL, NBA, MLB & Olympic Champion Athletes

INTRODUCTION

We all want a quick fix.

I used to want the same. I used to look at people who had purpose in their step, confidence in their bodies, and smiles on their faces and think, "I would give anything to be just like them." But I wasn't. Behind my smile were insecurities. Hidden masterfully beneath my all-American look and list of accomplishments were the heavy weights of self-doubt, the feeling of never being enough, and the pressure of perfectionistic thinking. A stranger might not have noticed; in fact, some of my closest friends would have been surprised at the thoughts I kept hidden behind my eyes. But they were there. Unbidden, unwanted, unneeded. For a long time I thought there was no other way to be. But I continued to watch.

When I noticed something helpful, I practiced it. I played with it. I took it and tried to make it my own. Some things fit, some things didn't. This book is a testament to the things that worked for me. I must admit, though, I didn't even have little successes until I started to give my thoughts to God. I started going to church more, reading His Word, and doing a better job of keeping up my end of the conversation with Him. Once my relationship with God started to heal, I noticed my insecurities with a more analytic mind; I could stand outside of myself and see the things that were really me and the things that I just thought were me. Most importantly, I saw confidence for what it truly was: a way of thinking given to us by God to empower us to have the courage to live the life He created us to live. That's when I began my detox from the insecurity that had been part of my daily diet, and that's what brought this book into existence.

If you've ever felt not enough, this book was written for you. If you've ever felt shackled by the chains of perfectionistic thinking, this book is for you. If you have ever been weighed down by self-doubt or insecurity, this book has been waiting for you to open it.

Friend, I am on this journey with you. If you picked up this book thinking it was an easy-to-swallow pill to reduce those thoughts that niggle at the back of your head—you are both right and wrong. You found a good pill, but it's going to be tough to swallow in one sitting.

Together we will swallow the detox pills—and do the work—to eliminate the weights on your soul. Your first prescription is to believe that there is a different way to think and live. For this detox to be effective, you must bring hope and belief for positive, lasting change, because change is possible, but it demands the right attitude in order to receive it.

My hope for you is that this book will inspire and motivate

you to challenge the status quo in your life. I built this book around the idea that confidence isn't just a personality trait; instead, it is a type of living. Confidence is a crucial component in what I refer to as *The Three M's*: mind, movement, and meaning—or in other words, your mental life, your physical life, and your spiritual life. Each detox section of this book is an examination of all three of these aspects. I apologize in advance if you were the kid who hated homework, because if you want to make lasting change, you have to practice new behaviors and new thoughts. As part of each chapter I include suggestions—assignments, really—just a swift kick in the butt, to move you from the toxic insecurities you live with every day, the insecurities that are keeping you from living your life to the absolute fullest.

Each detox section includes a brief discussion of the specific insecurity being detoxed and then three subset detoxes, all connected in theme, one each for your mind, body, and spirit. I recommend that you journey through this book slowly, taking one detox section per day so as not to rush your time for reflection and your ability to put the detox challenges into action. You may find that you need multiple days, or even a week, to fully complete and move through a detox section. Trust the pace that feels right for you.

I am confident that this cleanse, if fully adhered to, will transform the vocabulary of your mind, ridding you from the insecurities that have been holding you back and empowering you to conquer the life you have been given with confidence. May God bless you with true transformation that comes from the inside out.

EXPECTATIONS

The Truth: You only need to be you.

Instead of stretching and compressing yourself to become the person others think you should be, find the things that make your heart sing.

The Accordion Self

I've always had a thing for scraped knees. They were my childhood specialty. Every kid gets banged-up knees, but the kids with a streak of independence seem to get even more, and I was one of those kids. My mother says I came out of the womb wanting to do my own thing. When I first started walking, I spent my summer days teetering around the concrete pool deck while my older brother Nick played with friends in the water. As a result, I spent three months with knee pads to protect me from the countless, inevitable forward-tumbles I incurred daily. Undeterred, I was eager for my next stage of development so that I could seize even more freedom.

That stage came the year I discovered bicycles. I rode a tricked out, bubble-gum pink Schwinn classic with sparkly streamers on my handlebars. I was the coolest kid I knew.

Eventually, one summer I earned permission to cruise solo around the block with my best friend Kelly. We pedaled in our half-mile circle for hours on end, streamers flying, feeling like we owned the world. On Wednesdays, I bicycled with my brother a distance of three miles in the neighborhood to Mrs. Otsby's house for piano lessons.

The thing I most remember from my eight years of piano has nothing to do with piano and everything to do with scraped knees. I never liked the piano much, and I absolutely hated practicing my scales, but I did love the Wednesday afternoons Nick and I got to pedal back and forth to our lessons.

One memorable day, our music bag got stuck in the spokes of my wheels as I raced Nick down the hill from Mrs. Otsby's house. What ensued was a complex combination of somersaults and pavement rolls after I was thrown over my handlebars. I emerged from the tumble with bloody knees and gravel embedded deeply into my skin from my thighs down to my shins. We returned back to Mrs. Otsby's house, limping and bleeding into her immaculately kept home. I was never happier to see her than I was in that moment of need.

It's not that I didn't like Mrs. Otsby; it's just that I don't have a single musically inclined fiber in my body. Not only am I not musically talented, but I also don't like the process of music itself. Sure, I enjoy listening to and dancing to music, I just don't enjoy creating it, studying it, or playing it. Music just isn't my thing. It doesn't make my heart sing.

You know your heart is singing when you are able to lose yourself and in something you fully enjoy. For me, my heart sang when I rode my bike, swam in the pool, and wrote poems about the grass in our backyard.

But instead of embracing that, I spent years of my life stretching myself and then compressing myself to fit the mold of what I thought others expected of me. If my life were an instrument, it would be an accordion. Accordions elicit their harmonic sounds through a series of pulling and pushing, or compressing and expanding the instrument's bellows. And I pressed myself back and forth enough, contracting and expanding like an accordion in an attempt to meet the expectations of others' or society's often-unattainable ideals.

I also let other people press and pull me apart to play their song instead of my own. And since I let other people control the accordion handles, I never knew how to be my authentic self and how to play my own song. Have you ever struggled with this as well? As we journey through this constant battle of maximizing and minimizing ourselves with someone else controlling the song, it's no wonder that we are confused, downtrodden, and overwhelmed, wishing we could find peace with ourselves and with our life.

We have been told to live or act a certain way, to achieve certain things, or to want other things, yet at the very core of who we are, we just want to be ourselves. And the key to understanding our real identity is to understand our heart. We yearn for our hearts to sing, but we are so confined by the restrictions of others that we just don't know how.

When you know what makes your heart sing, and what brings out the music in your life, your life becomes a squeeze-box, emitting a melody and song as you go. Figuring out what makes your life sing is one of the first steps to claiming ownership over your personal identity.

For me, movement makes me come alive. Over the years, I have honed my listening skills and heard the song of my heart for movement, independence, and exploration. My song is composed of words, writing, foreign language, travel, adventure, running, snowboarding, photography, and the color pink. Separately, like musical notes out of sequence, these passions don't make a full song, but together, they compose a song of joy in the way I live.

When you take the time to think about what you love and about what comes naturally to you, you learn something valuable that can change the quality of your life when put into application. The things that make our heart sing are the intangibles, breathed into us by God, that express themselves visibly when we give them the opportunity to do so. When we sing the song God gave us, the invisible becomes visible, and beauty emanates.

Pick the accordion up; this time you're in control and it's your song that you are playing. It's time to give up the gig of expanding and compressing to fit the unpredictable expectations of the world around us; time to move the instrument of your life the way it was meant to move. The song you have been given to sing is unique to you, and you will know it by listening closely to the things that you naturally love to do. To learn how to be your best self—to play the instrument of your life well—you don't have to change. Rather, you simply need to be more of who you already are. Be a fully committed, loud version of you . . . scraped knees and all. Be "all in" with being who you are meant to be, take control of your personal accordion, and your song will be a masterpiece.

PHYSICAL DETOX
The New Rules of Wellness

A lot of people haven't found balance in their health and wellness; not for a lack of trying and effort, but rather for a lack of clear, simple, and correct information. The multibillion-dollar diet industry has preyed on the desperation of people seeking to implement positive physical habits in their lives, and as a result, an overabundance of contradicting advice, diets, and workouts exists.

Health and wellness can be much simpler than we've all made it out to be, and your first physical detox is intended to help you set the record straight for yourself. It's time to simplify the information. It's time to make reaching your optimal level of fitness and health realistically attainable to fit your lifestyle.

I have four basic tenants for you to follow from here on out. Let these be the pillars of your new approach to wellness, and let them guide you to make balanced and positive decisions about what you put into your body and how you take care of your body.

Rule #1: *Sleep More*

Sleep is one of the most underrated tenants of health and wellness. Sleep is actually an incredibly important component for successful weight loss and maintenance. The body performs its reparative functions during your sleep cycles. Furthermore, fulfilling your body's sleep requirements actually boosts your natural metabolic rate, ultimately helping you maintain a more consistent level of high energy and natural caloric burn.

Rule #2: *Stress Less*

Stress is a sneaky enemy that has become culturally accepted as a part of life. Not only is stress sneaky, but it also has the adverse physiological effect of releasing cortisol, also known as the stress hormone. When cortisol levels increase past their natural set point in the body, they store fat, particularly in the stomach region. So, if you want to have a flatter stomach and eliminate your love handles, eradicate stress from your life as much as you can. You can reduce your level of stress by cutting down your to-do list, by adding more sleep into your schedule, and by pursuing excellence, not perfection, in what you do.

Rule #3: *Eat More*

Opposite to popular opinion, the more you eat, the less you will actually weigh. In many cases, people who want to lose weight and severely restrict their caloric intake actually end up sabotaging themselves by forcing their bodies into what is commonly referred to as "starvation mode." When one's caloric intake is too low, the body holds on to extra fat for storage, ultimately slowing down one's natural metabolism. Extreme calorie restriction can promote quick weight loss. However, in most cases, it is weight that is immediately gained back because of the sabotaged metabolism. To boost your metabolism, your energy, and to promote maintenance of your ideal body weight, it is important to eat wholesome and nutritionally packed food frequently throughout the day.

Rule #4: *Move More*

The more you move your body, the more your body will be able to move. Being fit and active becomes easier to maintain once you have established movement as a regular part of your daily life. To move more, choose fitness activities that you enjoy— you will get the best results and you will be most consistent with exercise that you enjoy. There is no right or wrong way to exercise. Rather, there is a best way for each individual. Create a fitness and movement lifestyle that is a good fit for you and that you can implement and sustain in your day-to-day life.

MENTAL DETOX

The Lies in Your Mind

One of the reasons I wasted so many years as an accordion— changing myself to fit the mold dictated by those around me— is because I looked to the world around me to validate whether or not I was special or fit in. Anyone who sets out on a quest like this is certain to come back beaten down and heartbroken about themselves, and I believed the lie that I wasn't anything special. Since I didn't think I was special or that I had anything special to offer the world, I didn't listen to any internal wisdom that may have been coming from God.

I'm sure you've felt this way at some point in your life, too, that you weren't special or had nothing to offer. This foundational lie creates a plethora of other lies that we are then susceptible to believe. Lies like being *average,* being *not good enough,* being *fearful,* being *unlovable,* being *timid,* and being *forgettable.* We must choose to overcome this mindset and to stop playing the accordion with our lives by aggressively detoxing our thoughts, in particular, the thoughts we have about ourselves.

To work through this mental detox, first identify the top three most pervasive lies that have dominated your self-identity and write them down in the spaces provided below:

1) ....

2) ....

3) ....

Now, replace those three lies with opposite statements. These are the truths about who you are, even if you don't quite believe them to be true yet. For example, if one of the lies you wrote down in the space above was *"I am average and unnoticeable,"* then the truth you will write in the corresponding space below is *"I am special, noticeable, and have something great to give to others and to the world."*

1) ....

2) ....

3) ....

SPIRITUAL DETOX

Hearing the Song God Put on Your Heart

For we are God's masterpiece. He has created us anew in Christ Jesus, so we can do the good things he planned for us long ago. (Ephesians 2:10)

God made only one you. You are the only you to exist, in the present, in the past, or in the future. There is a reason God made you: your life—your song—gives Him great pleasure because it sings of His glory. That means that you have a unique song to sing, a song that has never been sung before and one that will never be sung again, so you must make sure it is sung.

To be the best version of yourself—that is, to fulfill your purpose—you must first get to know yourself. To get to know yourself you have to slow down, get quiet, and listen to the things about life that make your heart sing.

Your first spiritual detox is a self-reflective exercise to learn how to better hear the song God put on your heart and on your life. To do this, take ten minutes today to think intentionally about exactly what it is that you *love* to do. What are the things that make your soul sing? What would you do if you didn't have to work, run errands, or clean the house? Exactly what are the activities and things in which you can lose yourself and lose time while doing them, the things that make you feel engaged, creative, and alive?

Don't rush through making this list or underestimate the value of knowing what makes your heart come alive. Use the space below to come up with ten things you really enjoy doing, and if you aren't sure what you enjoy doing now, think about the things that you enjoyed doing as a child and list those:

1) ....

2) ....

3) ....

4) ....

5) ....

6) ....

7) ....

8) ....

9) ....

10) ....

....

Father, Help me hear the song You have sown into my heart, that I might learn to live with authenticity, being who You created me to be. Free me from the burden I feel to meet the expectations of others and show me how I can change my perspective to live only for Your approval, not for the approval of others. In the powerful name of Jesus, Amen.

EMOTIONAL BAGGAGE

The Truth: God has freed you from your past.

Whether your trash is self-doubt, insecurity, or a critical voice in your head, it's time to take your trash to the dump.

The Dump

I inherited a hard work ethic from my father. A union pipefitter who worked ten-hour shifts, he commuted two hours from our rural town in Virginia to Washington, D.C., and back every day. He parked his 1978 Ford just outside of my bedroom window, and every morning his headlights shined through as he left for the day. Half asleep, I always waved to him even though I knew he couldn't see me. Since the inconsistency of being in the construction business meant work was never guaranteed, when there was work, Dad would work. He never took weekends, vacations, or sick days. If there was work, he would work. Period.

Our quality time came on the occasional evening he got home early and on the rare weekend that he would have off.

Those weekends were filled with household chores and an inexhaustible honey-do list, but they were special because he allowed me to "help." I'm sure I got in the way more than I helped, but he made me feel irreplaceable. My favorite chore was the trip to the dump.

The dump meant we needed to load the bed of his rusty red truck with trash, leaves, and the like before taking the twenty-minute ride down country roads together. He would play classic rock and I would chat his ear off about my dolls, tea parties, and dreams. At the dump I got to stand on the truck bed and pass him item after item to add to the mountain of community trash tucked away behind the fenced walls. Sometimes he would let me chuck a light bag myself, allowing me to throw it as far as I could toward the deposit center. My throws never made it very far. Dad always picked the bag up and took it all the way for me. The satisfaction of emptying bag after bag until only stray leaves and small piles of dirt remained was cathartic. I loved how light the truck felt after we completed our chore. I also loved knowing how happy Mom would be when she saw us come back with an empty (and cleanish) truck.

We've all got trash, internal trash. It's baggage that weighs on our souls and it's heavy. We drag it around with us wherever we go and it burdens us. The problem is that we have gotten so used to the burden that we barely notice it; what we do notice is that something about our lives is just not quite right.

The trash that you carry hides in your thoughts. Your trash might be self-doubt or insecurity or it might be the critical or discouraging thing that someone in your past once said to you. Regardless of what your trash looks like, it's time to take it to the dump. Get rid of it.

In order to know our true selves—our true identity and who God created us to be—we must let go of the trash of our past. We are not defined by our past; rather, if we dump our trash, we can be refined by it.

Often we don't take our internal trash to the dump because we aren't sure where to even start. We want change, but change feels so distant that we resign ourselves to just staying the same and hope that eventually change will happen. The thing is, if you want something to change, you must first make a change. The good news is that change is easier than you think—in fact, you don't even have to know where the dump is to get yourself to the dump. All you need to do is jump into the truck with your trash loaded up and be a passenger. When you are willing to cleanse yourself of the baggage that has been weighing you down, God will drive you and direct you where you need to go to unload the junk you've accumulated. What's important is that you must first be willing to let it all go.

It is once we arrive at the dump—with a full awareness of what our trash actually is—that we stand on the edge of the truck bed and begin the process. We must initiate the cleanse. We must pick up bag after bag and be willing to toss it toward the dumping hole. We don't need to worry about how far we can throw our trash; we just need to be willing to throw it away from ourselves. In the same way my dad picked up my bags that had fallen short, so, too, does God pick up our baggage and take it the whole way once we decide to dispose of that which is weighing us down.

Crafted within you is a beautiful identity, uniquely placed in you by God. In order to see and live as the person you were created to be, you must take a trip to the dump.

Get rid of the baggage and trash that you have held on to from your past. Your past does not predict your future unless you let it. Your future is full of possibility and purpose—awaken that potential by embracing the person you were created to be.

PHYSICAL DETOX

Fridge Cleanse

To help you get into the mindset of dumping all of your trash, your physical detox is to literally clean out your refrigerator/freezer. This will not only cleanse your kitchen, but it will also help you feel empowered with momentum to continue the cleansing process of getting rid of trash in your life.

Throw out anything that is expired or that is not often used. Place the remaining items on your counter so you can wipe down the shelves and drawers of your refrigerator and freezer. Once your deep clean is complete, reload the items in an organized fashion.

If you are committed to optimizing your health and nutrition, you can take this fridge cleanse to the next level by trashing any item that has more than five ingredients listed on its packaging. Doing so will reduce your intake of manufactured and processed foods and will leave your refrigerator filled with whole, natural foods that are ideal for optimal health.

MENTAL DETOX
Purging Past Identities

Now that you have done a physical purge of your fridge, it's time to do a mental purge and begin dumping the trash in your mind.

If you believe in Jesus Christ, the old you is gone and only the new you exists. Consider the words of 2 Corinthians 5:17: "This means that anyone who belongs to Christ has become a new person. The old life is gone; a new life has begun!" Use the space below to write out five identifiers to describe the "old you." Select words or phrases that you have used in your mental self-talk to limit yourself or criticize yourself, words that are keeping you stuck in an old life when a new life is available to you:

....

....

....

....

....

These are now on paper. You have identified these toxic thoughts as trash. This is akin to loading the truck bed with bags of trash. Now you need to drive to the dump. Take the phrases above and mark them out with a dark pen or a Sharpie. This is equivalent to shredding a piece of trash. You are making these phrases obsolete from your life, your mind, and your vocabulary. They are no longer who you are and you no longer have permission to use them in your internal self-talk.

SPIRITUAL DETOX
His Opinion

The humble will see their God at work and be glad. Let all who seek God's help be encouraged. (Psalm 69:32)

God's opinion is the only opinion that matters. You are who He says you are. As you prepare today to dump the trash of your past, allow God to cleanse your perception of yourself. Pray that He would change your internal eyes to understand who He created you to be.

Here are just a few truths that God says about you:

> You are a child of God. (John 1:12)
> You are fearfully and wonderfully made. (Psalm 139:14)
> You are a friend of Jesus. (John 15:15)
> You have been cleansed and redeemed. (Romans 3:24)
> You are forgiven. (Ephesians 1:7)
> You are no longer slave to sin and trash. (Romans 8:1)
> You are free. (Galatians 5:1)
> You are blessed. (Ephesians 1:3)
> You are chosen. (Ephesians 1:4)
> You are taken care of by God. (Philippians 4:19)
> You are more than a conqueror. (Romans 8:37)
> You are not alone. (Hebrews 13:5)

You are not helpless. (Philippians 4:13)
You are promised a full life. (John 10:10)
You are secure. (Ephesians 2:20)
You have hope. (Ephesians 1:12)
You have purpose. (Ephesians 1:9)
You have strength. (Ephesians 6:10)
You are victorious. (1 Corinthians 15:57)
You are a light in this world. (Matthew 5:14)

....

Father, I am weary from carrying my emotional baggage everywhere I go and I am ready to give it over to You. Take my burdens and my insecurities from me. Teach me how to dump the lies of my mind and how to replace them with the truth about who I really am and about how much You love me. In the loving name of Jesus, Amen.

OLD PATTERNS

The Truth: Your thoughts can be trained.

Old thought patterns sabotage your future. It's time to lay new tracks in your brain and change your destination.

The Train in Our Brain

In 1987, trains became a staple in the Blackwell household. That Christmas my older brother Nick received a Lionel model train set from Santa Claus. The set was so elaborate and expansive that it took up our entire guest bedroom. Its tracks wove in and out of an entire plastic model village and the engine revved with the lights and sounds of a real locomotive. Nick was always the train conductor, but I got to watch and be in charge of the fake village people and the narrative of the story we acted out.

I followed Nick's fascination with trains to Europe, as he was the first to travel to and live there. The stories of his train adventures did not disappoint and I soon found myself riding the rails through Europe. Those train tracks transported me to new horizons. I can still remember the very first time I caught a glimpse of the Swiss Alps. I had just woken up from a nap, and as my eyes opened, my heart skipped a beat. I jumped out of my seat, compelled by wonder, and pressed my face against the window. The beauty was greater than I could have ever previously imagined. That day, with that first peek at the peaks of the Swiss Alps, the frame of reference with which I saw the world expanded. My internal mental tracks were being re-railed.

Each new track I traveled led me to newfound personal revelations and delights. As I traveled from country to country I saw thousands of tracks and rail intersections, each with numerous possibilities of direction and destination. In the same way, our brains are complex highways of neuron tracks crisscrossing and intersecting. There is a train in our brain fueled by our thoughts with thousands of track intersections that direct our actions and ultimately our futures.

Imagine every thought you have ever had as a railroad track. Whatever thoughts you have allowed yourself to dwell on have, over time, become the routes of preference for your neurological train. If you want to change the destination your mental train takes, you need to reconstruct the layout of the tracks. And more than just changing the tracks, you need to run the new tracks over and over again to set them concretely into place. As Henry David Thoreau wrote, "As a single footstep will not make a path on the earth, so a single thought will not make a pathway in the mind. To make a deep physical path, we walk again and again. To make a deep mental path, we must think over and over the kind of thoughts we wish to dominate our lives."

To reconstruct our internal tracks we must define the

route by thinking over and over again on the right thing. Applying this type of focused mindset is how new rails are staked to the ground.

In addition to the laying down of new track, you may need to disable old tracks that were taking you in the wrong direction. The tracks of insecurity that lie in our minds are deeply ingrained, but they do not have to stay that way. You can disable those tracks by changing the vocabulary of your mind. Once you remove these railroad ties—any negative, self-limiting, or self-doubting thoughts—you can stop taking the tracks of insecurity.

Your brain is under construction, and like all construction, it takes time to build and rebuild. As you uproot your old tracks and lay down the new ones for your neurological train to follow, keep in mind that your internal dialogue determines your destination. Every thought you have matters. Every time you capture an old thought—or old track—and reframe it into a new one makes a difference. Every small step toward positive change is worthy of celebration. The words that you say to yourself affect everything you do, how you see the world, and how you live. The words you use construct your world.

In the same way that Nick and I used to uproot and then reroute the Lionel train tracks with new routes, you, too, have control over how your mental tracks are laid out. You are the master architect and conductor of your thoughts—and your thoughts won't change themselves, they need your direction. Lay out new tracks and you will find yourself staring out at unexpected and breathtaking mountain peaks on your new route in life.

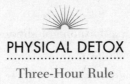

PHYSICAL DETOX
Three-Hour Rule

One of the most effective ways to stay on track with your healthy eating habits is to eat small, frequent meals throughout the day. Following the Three-Hour Rule—that is, eating something small every three hours—will help you remember to stay on track with a healthy eating schedule.

Imagine that your metabolism is like a steam-powered locomotive. It is a powerful train that you need to keep feeding—or burning coal to create the steam—in order to keep the engine going. So, too, is your metabolism. The more frequently you feed it—or eat—the more powerful the engine will be—or, in other words, the more elevated your metabolic rate will be. The higher your metabolic rate is, the higher your natural caloric burn at rest will be, meaning that you will naturally stay lean and fit. Additionally, the higher your metabolism, the more naturally energetic you will feel.

Below are some suggestions of small, healthy snacks to eat as you implement the Three-Hour Rule and thereby boost your metabolism:

- An apple with a tablespoon of peanut butter or almond butter
- A whey protein shake
- A prepackaged protein bar
- A handful of unsalted raw almonds
- Baby carrots and hummus
- Celery sticks with peanut butter

- A banana
- Rice cake with a teaspoon of almond butter
- Walnuts or pistachios
- Baked chickpeas
- Hard-boiled eggs
- Edamame beans, fresh or dried
- Slices of lean deli turkey with a slice of Swiss cheese
- Low-fat cottage cheese
- Greek yogurt

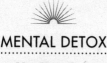

MENTAL DETOX
Not Your Past

As you work toward deepening the grooves of your new tracks you must remember not to be derailed by the tracks of your past that beckon to you. Many of us struggle with staying on our new tracks because we've spent years, possibly even decades, convincing ourselves that we are defined and beholden to our past. You are not your past; your past does not define you, it refines you.

To help you gather up new positive rails to put your past into perspective as you work on the reconstruction of your mind, below are some truths about the place of your past:

Your past is behind you.
Your past has brought you to where you are.
Your past has refined you.

Your past has created a story that only you can tell.
Your past allows you to empathize more authentically
   with others.
Your past gives you the ability to need grace.
Your past is not your present.

Recognize the words of your past—from yourself and from others—and categorize them properly. Put the past in its proper place by refusing to let it weigh you down any longer. Your past does not belong in your present, and it certainly doesn't belong in your future. Stop allowing the past to haunt you; it is over and you are free to walk burden-free into your present and future.

SPIRITUAL DETOX

Defining God

Give thanks to the Lord, for He is good! His faithful love endures forever. (Psalm 107:1)

In the same way that you may have lived with unhealthy train tracks in your brain about who you think you are, you very well might have decrepit tracks about who you think God is. For this spiritual detox, cleanse your understanding of God by making sure you have an accurate definition of who He is. First, think for a few minutes about who you think God is and who He has been to you. Now, take that definition and compare it to what the Bible tells us about God:

God is good. (Psalm 119:65–72)

God is love. (1 John 4:7–10)

God is infinite. (Romans 11:33)

God is all powerful. (Jeremiah 32:17)

God is unchanging. (Psalm 102:25–28)

God is just. (Psalm 75:1–7)

God is holy. (Revelation 4:8–11)

God is everywhere. (Psalm 139:7–12)

God is all knowing. (Psalm 139:1–6)

God is merciful. (Deuteronomy 4:29–31)

God is wise. (Proverbs 3:19–20)

God is faithful. (Psalm 89:1–8)

God is Father. (Romans 8:15–17)

God is transcendent. (Psalm 113:4–5)

....

Father, You are so good. I praise You and thank You for helping me change the old patterns in my life. Thank You for walking alongside me as I lay down new tracks and a new way of living. In the hopeful name of Jesus, Amen.

NEGATIVE SELF-TALK

The Truth: Your thoughts have power.

Ditch the self-defeating tunes in your head and upgrade to life-giving thoughts.

Upgrade Your Walkman

As a child, what did you want to be when you grew up? I always wanted to be a professional ice skater. My childhood musical tastes revolved around music appropriate for the choreographed carpet-skating routines I designed in the privacy of my bedroom, aided by the accompaniment of my boom box: Ace of Base, Whitney Houston, Jem and the Holograms, and No Doubt. I played these old tapes over and over in the privacy of my room long after cassettes became obsolete and were replaced by CDs. My parents had given me a Discman, which I used in public so other kids would think I was cool, but every night I went home to my boom box and my tapes.

We all have old tapes. They are familiar and comforting soundtracks that get rewound and listened to over and over again. Somewhere in the repetition the message fades into the background of unquestionable truth. These tapes are not only outdated but the information they contain themselves needs to be upgraded. In public we act as if we are cool and collected—a façade that we have it all together—and in private we go back home to the comfort of our old tapes in the comfort of our minds.

There are many types of old tapes, but most often our old tapes are the negative things others have said about us, the fears we have come to know intimately, and the names we call ourselves. These old tapes are the thoughts that we have always come to accept as true because they have always been part of our subconscious thoughts and of the internal dialogue we have. We are so used to them that it is sometimes difficult to distinguish that they are there in the first place, which is why we often don't realize what we allow them to play in our ears and say to us. It is imperative that we pull these tapes out of the basement of our brain. We must clean them out, but to do that, we need to know how to identify what needs to go and what can stay.

The dangerous thing about the autoplay of the tapes in our minds is that we don't always really hear the words that are being spoken. In the same way that I didn't pay attention to the lyrics in the songs that set the stage for my carpet-skating routines, we often don't listen closely enough to the songs and words that play in our minds. We don't realize that we have been listening to song after song on repeat without actually taking the time to notice the lyrics. Words are perhaps the most powerful responsibility we are ever given, as they have the power of life or death over our lives. There is no such thing as a word, or string of words, having a neutral effect upon our brains. They either build us up, or they tear us down. The words we hear ultimately become the words we speak, and the words we speak to ourselves about ourselves—that is, our thoughts—matter more than we could possibly comprehend.

It is time for you to ditch the tapes—and the CDs while you're at it—and upgrade to MP3s in your thinking. Like any technological product, your thoughts will always demand attention and upgrading to stay up to date and at maximum capacity. Our ability to think and choose our own thoughts is more powerful than any technological advancement, so we need to train and choose our thoughts with intention.

Change the autoplay in your mind by picking words that speak life:

- I am unique and was created for a purpose.
- I am already good enough because I am me.
- My body is beautiful.
- I am a conqueror.
- I am blessed and live in abundance.
- I am becoming the right person and will eventually meet the right person.
- I am well-loved and well-appreciated.
- I am confident and I will continue to choose to be that way.
- I trust my decisions and myself.
- I'm worth it.
- I can do it. I can do anything.
- Every small step of progress I make toward a goal matters.
- I am likable because I am my true self.

- I always follow through.
- I am gifted in the areas I am meant to be.
- The only thing expected of me is to try my best each and every day.
- My opinion matters greatly and I have good ideas.
- I am growing, developing, and transforming each and every day.
- I am smart and am getting smarter every day.
- God has promised to not give me more than I can handle.

Take the boom box off your shoulder, ditch the cassette tape you've been listening to on repeat, and use phrases like the examples above to upgrade your internal dialogue. Each time you do you are speaking words of life to yourself that will continually upgrade your mind, making it better and better each and every day it stays up to date. Create a soundtrack of praise and gratitude to accompany your life and your soul will sing.

PHYSICAL DETOX
New Exercise Tapes

One of the old tapes that I had on repeat for way too many years was my motivation behind exercising. I was obsessed with exercise strictly for calorie burn and weight control. My tape was challenged by one of my best friends, Moe, a personal trainer. She approaches exercise as an opportunity to invest in the longevity of her life. Every day she asked herself if the movement she did would help her live happily and healthily into her nineties. Moe celebrates her "good" workout days and her "bad" ones equally because she doesn't believe in good or bad, but rather just in celebrating the fact that she has invested in and honored her body through movement.

Using Moe's wisdom as a guide, upgrade your internal tape on exercise by reprogramming the purpose behind why you are motivated to work out. This week treat yourself to variety; buy a few new songs to listen to while you walk, run, or workout. Also, try listening to a few podcast shows that are new to you—you might find that listening to the right podcast host will make you feel like you are exercising with a friend. I would love to be your company and help you celebrate the opportunity to move—allow me to join you by listening to my iTunes podcast show *Confidence on the Go,* which you can access free in iTunes or at www.trishblackwell.com/podcasts.

You know, of course, that working out has myriad benefits such as stress relief, better sleep, and improved cardiovascular health. But it goes far beyond that: exercise can prevent injury, balance your hormones, accelerate brain function, and improve your sex drive. By viewing exercise with this positive lens you will find yourself successful in your fitness commitments, but more importantly happy as you move your body in enjoyment.

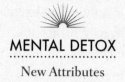

MENTAL DETOX
New Attributes

To upgrade your mental tapes you simply have to decide to think differently and with more intention. Each time you change or substitute a thought, you are upgrading your software—or changing from a cassette tape to an MP3 file.

As you consider the internal tapes you have allowed to play in the background of your life, try to identify the three tapes that seem to be the most familiar to you or that play the loudest and write them in the space provided on the next page. To help you as you reflect on this exercise, some examples of common old tapes are phrases and beliefs such as:

- I am average; and all I'll ever be is average.
- I am never going to be good enough.
- I am ugly and no one will ever think I'm beautiful.
- I am destined to struggle; life is hard and I will never catch a break.
- We will never have enough money.
- I will never meet the right person.
- No one appreciates me.
- No matter what I do, it's wrong.
- I'm not worth it.
- I can't do it.
- There's no use.
- People don't like me and won't like me.
- I never follow through.

- Other people are better and more talented than
  I am.
- I must be perfect.
- My opinion doesn't matter.
- I'll always be this way.
- I'm a fraud and everyone knows it.
- No one really likes me; they just pity me.
- If I were smarter I wouldn't be in this situation.

My old tapes:

1) ....

2) ....

3) ....

Taking the above list, start updating your internal mind-set by rewriting those statements. Take the negative, limiting phrase and position it in a positive way.

My new tapes:

1) ....

2) ....

3) ....

Next, as you continue upgrading your internal dialogue, write out the five major characteristics you want to describe your life. By identifying these attributes you will be able to position them at the forefront of your mind, thereby changing the internal atmosphere of your thoughts.

To assist you as you contemplate these five character traits for your new mental MP3 files, here are a few suggestions: confidence, power, action, inspirational, successful, beauty, intelligence, congruency, authenticity, happiness, honesty, kindness, love, hope, and positivity.

The five character traits I claim:

1) ....
2) ....
3) ....
4) ....
5) ....

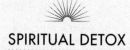

SPIRITUAL DETOX
Upgrade with God

The Lord passed in front of Moses, calling out "Yahweh! The Lord! The God of compassion and mercy! I am slow to anger and filled with unfailing love and faithfulness. I lavish unfailing love to a thousand generations. (Exodus 34:6–7)

In terms of our spiritual walks, we each journey through varying stages of development in our relationship to and understanding of God. Equally important to our understanding the character of God is our understanding of how He sees us. Upgrade your confidence of core identity by writing a letter from God's perspective to you, as His child. Start the letter by writing one or two sentences about how much He loves you; next, write one or two sentences about how beautiful He thinks the character of your heart has become; and finish with one or two sentences about the future of positive change He has planned for you.

Dear Child,

....

....

....

....

....

....

....

Love,
God, your Father

....

> *Father, thank You for helping me see myself as*
> *You see me. I fervently pray that You continue*
> *to break the chains of negative self-talk and low*
> *self-esteem that have kept me shackled to the*
> *sidelines of life. Open my mind and my heart*
> *to really believe in the truth of who I am in You*
> *and teach me how to see myself through Your*
> *eyes. In the beautiful name of Jesus, Amen.*

TRYING TO BE SOMEONE ELSE

The Truth: You are unique.

Celebrate your God-breathed passions and be in tune to how God loves you through the quirks that make you unique.

Chocolate Peanut Butter and Edamame Beans

I always wanted a bunny when I was a little girl, but my parents limited our family pets to dogs and cats. This bunny obsession put the Easter Bunny, along with Bugs Bunny or any rabbit for that matter, high up in my esteem. Even though I was raised to celebrate Easter around the true reason for the season—the resurrection of Christ—I admittedly always looked forward to the Easter Bunny more than the holiday itself, even when I was too old to believe in the Easter Bunny or the magical eggs he brings.

Even as an adult I don't consider myself too old for an Easter basket and love the tradition of exchanging baskets with my husband. He obliges purely to satiate my excitement.

Our Easter baskets reflect just how different we each are.

Brandon's overflows with every variation of Reese's peanut butter chocolate possible and a few car deodorizers for his Jeep. Mine is filled with nut mixes, edamame beans, sugar-free gum, Listerine, and hair ties. There is nothing about his basket that entices me and he feels the same about mine. We have different tastes, different preferences, and different interpretations of what we each consider an Easter "treat."

Beyond the Reese's Cups and edamame beans, we each have quirks that are hard to explain away. I stop everything I am doing any time I hear French being spoken. Brandon learns Japanese while watching anime cartoons on Saturdays. I thrive off a regimented schedule and to-do list and Brandon walks through life without an agenda. I can't stand it when my mouth doesn't feel clean—so I keep Listerine or gum in practically every room in my house as well as in my car. Brandon is passionate about keeping the environment clean and will walk a mile to recycle an aluminum can. I recycle only because I feel guilty if I don't. We are both odd-balls in our own right, and to be honest, I believe that we all are. It is these quirks that make us so complex and so utterly unique; these are the things about ourselves worthy of celebration.

You are worthy of celebration because you were created in the image of God. More than that, God handcrafted you—every aspect of you—with intention and specificity. There is only one you. Woven into your heart are the workings of a complex web of uniqueness that only you possess. This tapestry is a combination of your talents and traits. The threads are vibrant and eclectic, yet seamlessly work together to create an imprint of personality that only you can impress upon the world. Simply put, there is a reason why you love what you love. There is a reason why you are good at what you are good at. There is a reason why you look the way you do. There is a reason why your story is your story. God wove the threads of your life with a personality, gifts, and quirks that are only found in you. And even though they may not make sense as a whole to you, they do to Him.

In the same way that you care about the ones you love, God, too, cares about everything you care about. In fact, our God is a God who takes great pleasure in shining His love down on us; and often this is done in the silence and simplicity of the little things.

This pleasure is unveiled through the way He speaks to our quirks. To speak to me He sends me bunnies that skirt along my path, making me smile. He paints the sky with my favorite array of pinks and purples to rope my heart to His. He blesses me with friends who are generous in their love and in their gifting of dark sea salt chocolate and bottles of Malbec.

To know and feel this love that God is already showering around you, you must first understand what you love. It's easy to miss God in the small things if you aren't paying attention to the right things. God is serenading you, but to hear Him you need to let your heart be free to engage openly in the loves that come so naturally to you.

The little things that make your heart sing—and the quirks that make you, you—are actually big things. They are foundational to your personality and are instrumental to helping you fully live out the story that God has planned for you. Celebrate your quirks; you have them for a reason and you never know what rabbit hole they will take you down. The more we learn to live out the uniqueness that's been placed within us, the more free to be ourselves we will learn to be.

The more we allow our true selves to shine, the more impact our lives can and will have.

PHYSICAL DETOX
Sugar Slash

The most significant difference distinguishing my Easter basket from my husband's is the amount of sugar stuffed into the items placed so gingerly in those small wicker baskets. Sugar is perhaps the most insidious culprit in the decline of health, and it is sneaky. Hidden in practically every processed food product, sugar is not only toxic to our health, but addictive as well. The average American diet contains more than 80 grams of sugar per day, double the recommended daily allotment (RDA) of 40 grams per day advised by the U.S. Department of Agriculture (USDA).

Sugar has many clever aliases: honey, maltodextrin, malt syrup, mannitol, molasses, refiner's syrup, sorbitol, sorghum syrup, sucrose, grape sugar, golden syrup, fructose, high-fructose corn syrup, glucose solids, fruit juice, fruit juice concentrate, ethyl maltol, dextran, dextrose, corn syrup, corn syrup solids, date sugar, caramel, barley malt, turbinado sugar, and yellow sugar.

And it is well hidden in the following foods, which all rank high in sugar content: white bread, pastas, white rice, white flour, potatoes, corn, bananas, jams, salad dressings, fruit drinks, and alcohol.

Do a self-assessment today and write down everything you ate and drank yesterday. Now look up the sugar content for

each item you have listed by using the USDA's National Nu-
trient Database for Standard Reference website: http://ndb.
nal.usda.gov. Once you have determined how many grams of
sugar you currently intake, take the next three days to try to
whittle down your total sugar, with the goal of slashing your
sugar in half by the end of the three-day period.

MENTAL DETOX
Three Gifts

The key to understanding our hearts is found in acknowledging, and thereby unlocking, the gifts that we hold within
us. Combined, these gifts are what make your soul so beautiful and so unique. Resist the temptation to undersell your
strengths or compare your gifts to those of others. Your gifts,
just like your heart, are individual to you.

Take a few minutes to reflect and decide exactly what your
greatest three personal gifts are, writing them in the space provided below. Think about your strengths, about what comes
naturally to you, and about what others tend to compliment
you on as insight to what your three gifts are. Keep in mind
that you have more than three gifts, but for the sake of this
exercise we are simply going to highlight your greatest gifts so
you can better understand yourself and your heart.

Gift #1: ....

Gift #2: ....

Gift #3: ....

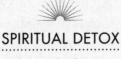

SPIRITUAL DETOX
God-Breathed Passion

But our bodies have many parts, and God has put each part just where he wants it. How strange a body would be if it had only one part! Yes, there are many parts, but only one body. The eye can never say to the hand, "I don't need you." The head can't say to the feet, "I don't need you." In fact, some parts of the body that seem weakest and least important are actually the most necessary. (1 Corinthians 12:18–22)

As you know, there is purpose behind the things in your heart that make you come alive. Like a necessary part of the body, God created you with specific abilities to contribute to the rest of the world, or body. These interests, passions, and pursuits are God-breathed, and even if they don't make sense to you, embrace them.

Study your heart today. As you reflect upon what you love to do and what captivates your attention and interest, pick one thing that really makes your heart sing. This one thing should be something you so enjoy that you lose track of time when thinking about it or doing it. It is an interest or pursuit that makes your spirit soar and excites you to be engaged in life.

Once you have identified one of your God-breathed passions, use the space on the next page to make a list of the specific reasons *why* you love that thing. The more detailed you are the better. Let your mind just free-flow with descriptions and explanations of what it is about that thing that you love so much. This exercise is meant to help you extract even more appreciation out of what you love and to help you become more attuned to the workings of your heart.

....

....

....

....

....

....

....

....

....

Father, thank You for making me who I am. Teach me how to be myself, how to be the person You created me to be that I might become a beautiful reflection of Your glory and Your love. Help me identify when I am trying to imitate others and give me the courage to be the unique person You intended me to be. In the bold name of Jesus, Amen.

UNWORTH

The Truth: You are good enough.

You are completely worthy of love simply because God's love bestows worth on you, and not because of your goodness.

You're Never Halfway Pregnant

I remember everything about that pee. I peed onto that stick, capped it, set it on the bathroom sink counter, and proceeded to pace around the house for exactly three minutes. Three minutes is a long time to wait for life-changing news. Heart racing, I picked the test back up. One small piece of plastic was about to tell me my future.

Two faint pink lines stared back at me.

Or at least that's what I thought. One of the lines was faded. I couldn't tell what it meant. Were there two lines or was it just one line and a half faded one? The difference between two lines and one line designated life inside of me or not. I ran to the kitchen, downed a bottle of water, and pulled out a new test.

An eternity of life seemed to pass during those next minutes of waiting. Teetering on the edge of parenthood I just wanted to know what the lines meant. I needed to know if I was really pregnant or not at all. The uncertainty made me feel like I was halfway between both states. I thought about my childhood, my adolescence, my parents, my travels, my husband, our wedding, and our hopes and dreams for a family. Another three minutes passed.

Two pink lines.

I *was* pregnant.

My body started shaking. Tears streamed down my face. It was clear my hormones had already started kicking in because the tears took me by surprise. I thought I'd be cool, calm, and eager to tell my husband. Instead I was the opposite: nervous, overwhelmed, uncontrollably joyful, and absolutely unable to express myself. I spent the rest of the day at work with my lips sealed and my mind running in circles. I bought a book on fatherhood from Barnes & Noble to gift to Brandon as a means of announcement and felt guilty all day carrying the secret of the baby around without him knowing.

To say that Brandon was elated is an understatement. He ran around the house in circles. Literally. Once he ran out of energy he then wanted to call everyone he knew to share his joy.

The next few weeks I was a ball of nerves. The joy of being pregnant was so wonderful that I was afraid it would be taken away from me, or really that I had misread the pink pregnancy test lines. That faded line made me so uncertain, as if I were stuck in the space between the two lines. As a result, every few days I convinced myself that I wasn't actually pregnant and I began purchasing pregnancy tests in bulk. This anticipatory worry continued until our first doctor appointment where we finally got to hear our little Ellie's heartbeat and see her tiny body on the sonogram. I *was* actually pregnant. Like, all the way.

Like pregnancy, being good enough is never a halfway sort of thing. You are either pregnant or you are not. Similarly, you are either good enough or you are not. And yet, most of us spend our lives unsure of whether we are good enough or whether we are destined to fail. We exist waiting for someone to pull us out from in between the lines. We have convinced ourselves that to matter—to really be good enough to be noticed and special—is something that is earned and not innate. And so we hustle. We hustle for love, for accolades, and for acceptance, all in an effort to be enough.

The thing is, you are already good enough simply because you were created by God and are completely loved by Him. There is nothing to prove and no need to earn "being enough," because in His eyes you already are.

In other words, you are not halfway to being who you need to be. Rather, you are *already* who you need to be. You are good enough because God said you are. You are cleansed from sin because Jesus died for you. You are who you are meant to be, and the only risk you have of being only half-enough is if you don't believe the truth of who God says you are. As you see your worth through God's eyes, you will see that second pink line of life appear. And I believe that when you see those two pink lines in yourself, God rejoices like a man learning he has become a father.

PHYSICAL DETOX
....
Wake Up Shake Up

The *Wake Up Shake Up* is one of the best ways to start your day and set yourself up for success physically. It is a method you can use daily to invest in connecting with your body. As you feel more attune to yourself physically you will learn to embrace your body as being good enough as it is today. It takes just five minutes per day and consists of three "must do" moves. You can do the *Wake Up Shake Up* at any time of the day, but it is most effective when done first thing in the morning right after getting out of bed.

The basic *Wake Up Shake Up* goes as follows:

- 5 Sun Salutations
- 1-Minute Plank Hold
- 25 Air Squats

Below is a detailed explanation of these must-do moves:

Move #1: *The Sun Salutation*

In the sun salutation, the synchronization of the motion of your breath with the movement of your body is very important. In short, the motion of breathing is what drives the movement of the body into, through, and out of each of the poses in the sequence. Take your time with your poses, and always start with this as your must-do first move.

Start from a standing position. Inhale deeply, then exhale. Slowly raise your arms wide and then high over your head in a

sweeping motion as you inhale deeply again. On your next exhale, float your arms down, palms facing away from you and go
slowly into a forward fold with your body. Inhale and exhale
from your folded position, allowing your hands to hang toward
the ground and your head toward your knees, which can be
straight or slightly bent. Inhale and flatten your back into a
half-standing position, keeping your back flat like a tabletop,
with your arms dangling toward the ground, and then allowing
yourself to go back into the forward fold on your next exhale.
Bend your knees slightly and allow your hands to meet the
ground. Step one foot backward into a lunge position and then
bring the next one out, bringing your body into a full plank
position. Lower your body to the ground slowly, then, gently
exhaling into a cobra position, raise your chest off the ground
while keeping your hips and legs rested. Inhale and move
backward into a triangle, or downward dog position. To modify,
go into child's pose, with arms extended and hips resting on
your feet. Stay here for two breaths and then return to plank
position. From plank position, lunge the opposite leg forward
back under your body, and then gently bring in your other leg,
bringing your body to a forward fold position again. Inhale
slowly and then exhale your breath as you rise, one vertebrae at
a time, with your knees slightly bent, and elongate your body
with arms reaching as high above your head as possible.

Repeat your sun salutations as slowly as you desire, doing
at least 3 to 5 total salutations.

Move #2: *The Plank Hold*

This move is simple in demonstration and application. The
plank hold requires total body engagement and will shape your

shoulders, arms, core, and legs. In particular, the plank hold is highly effective for working the entire core, which is the abdominal wall and lower back region.

To execute the move, simply make your body parallel to the ground and lift yourself up on your toes and hands (an optional modification is to rest on your forearms instead of your hands). Make your body horizontal to the ground and strive to keep your body, from shoulders to hipbones, in alignment like a table. Essentially, you are putting your body into a push-up position, with your arms extended, and then not moving from there. You will be surprised at how effectively this stationary holding exercise works your entire body.

Hold the plank hold as long as you can, focusing on internally pulling your belly button toward your spine. Start by doing the plank hold for 20 to 30 seconds at a time if you are a beginner and work up to holding your plank position for 60 seconds without breaking, after which you can continue progressing your way to longer and longer holds. This is a move anyone can do and get great results, from the beginner exerciser to the elite athlete.

Move #3: *Air Squats*

The air squat needs no equipment and is an exercise you can do anywhere, even in your office or in a bathroom stall.

For a beginner, use your arms to swing and counterbalance you as you squat down. Pretend you are squatting down to hover over the toilet and then stand back up. Focus on hinging from the hips, keeping your knees over your ankles and focusing on pushing your butt backward and out. Do 25 total squats in whatever sequence of number you wish.

People with an intermediate fitness level can take the air squat up a notch by keeping their hands on their head (don't interlock your fingers, however, and resist the temptation to pull on your neck). Keep your hands on your head and shoot for a total number of 100 repetitions.

If you are advanced, do jump squats, the advanced version of air squats, jumping off the ground with each repetition. Jump squats are high-intensity calorie burners, so shoot for 3 to 5 sets of 15 to 20 reps to get your metabolism really revved.

For pictures of exactly what each must-do move looks like, download your free copy of the *Wake Up Shake Up* routine at www.trishblackwell.com/wakeup.

MENTAL DETOX

The Good Enough Challenge

For the next seven days, commit to the mental challenge of attacking any "not enough" thoughts that enter your mind. Typically these thoughts will arise when we are engaged in a comparison, when we are being self-critical, when we are pursuing perfectionism, or when we just feel overwhelmed and overscheduled. Whenever the sentiment of "not being enough" pops into your thoughts, catch it and throw it out. Replace it immediately with the following simple statement:

I am enough.

Simply thinking *I am enough* might not be proactive enough for cognitive replacement. Be intentional about saying the phrase out loud, and, if possible, take a piece of paper and write the sentence out a few times as well. Taking on this mental detox doesn't mean that you won't have these nagging negative and self-doubting thoughts, so don't be discouraged when you do. This detox is intended to help you actively choose to believe the truth that you are good enough as you are today. By carefully guarding your mind over the next seven days you are coating your confidence with an assurance that you are exactly who you are meant to be. You were created by God, who does not make mistakes, and that truth alone qualifies you as being "enough."

SPIRITUAL DETOX
Thanking God

Give thanks to the Lord and proclaim his greatness. Let the whole world know what he has done. (Psalm 105:1)

Use the following list to guide yourself in a daily prayer of gratitude to God, thanking Him for who and how He made you. Pray over these truths about who you are.

You are complete in Him. (Colossians 2:10)
You are free. (John 8:36)
You have the peace of God that passes all understanding. (Philippians 4:7)
You are lacking in nothing. (Philippians 4:9)
You can do anything. (Philippians 4:13)

You are an overcomer. (Revelation 12:11)

You are chosen. (1 Peter 2:9)

You are forgiven. (Ephesians 1:7)

You are filled with power, love, and a sound mind.
(2 Timothy 1:7)

You are backed and supported by God. (Romans
8:31)

You are perfectly made. (Psalm 139:14)

You are the apple of God's eye. (Psalm 17)

....

Father, help me understand my worth in Your eyes. Open my heart to my identity in You, that I might live free from feelings of unworthiness. In the worthy name of Jesus, Amen.

CONTROL

The Truth: You are loved.

Experience the ultimate soul cleanse by letting God do the work, and letting His love free you to play your beautiful part in the story of the world.

Detergent for the Soul

I was single when I purchased my first house. The investment represented a new phase of my maturity and personal growth and I was eager to establish myself as a responsible home-owner. My parents supported my purchase by gifting me a top-of-the-line washer and dryer set as a congratulatory gift.

After a few months of living alone, I opened my home up to friends who needed rooms to rent. After a few months, one of my roommates asked to borrow some laundry detergent because she had run out. I generously obliged and told her that it was just above the washer/dryer. She looked and said there was nothing there. Certain of my supply, I insisted that there was some and pulled my detergent off the shelf. She looked at me, shook her head, and asked for the detergent again.

As it turns out, I had handed her fabric softener. Forcing it on her again as detergent, she finally laughed and jokingly asked me if I knew the difference between detergent and softener. I actually didn't. I had been washing my clothes for months with fabric softener, and not detergent. I thought my clothes didn't seem optimally clean, but to be fair, I simply didn't know any better. I went to the only college in the country that included a full-scale laundry service. For four years I simply dropped off my bag of dirty clothes at the laundry hall and then received them back the next day, folded and pressed.

My clothes hadn't been getting clean, not because something was wrong with my washer or because my clothes were stained and old, but because I wasn't using the right supplies.

Similarly, we often use the wrong supplies in life without even knowing it.

Convinced by our upbringing and by society, we clean ourselves and establish our self-worth by furiously seeking approval, affirmation, and achievement. In the same way that fabric softener is not a replacement for detergent, so, too, is our effort to prove ourselves worthy not a substitute for having the peace that comes with knowledge of who we really are.

The only detergent that will clean your soul, and free you to be the person you were created to be, is God's truth that you are enough. Not only are you enough, you are more than enough: you were created with greatness in mind—it is a greatness meant to shine His glory. This greatness that God planted inside of us is uniquely displayed in each of our lives, according to the plan God has for our life. For some, greatness means parenting in such a way that it changes an entire generation. For others it means being instrumental in an organization that impacts those in poverty and need. For you it might mean writing a book that inspires others, leading a volunteer rally, mentoring a teenager, inviting your neighbors to church, helping the homeless, creating a business that positively influences your community, having a home that overflows with hospitality, or being an advocate for the environment. You have certain talents, interests, and innate abilities for a reason, and most likely, you are nowhere near tapping into your full potential. In the same way we are only able to see the tip of an iceberg, we can only see a small percentage of who we really are deep down. The submerged portion of our identity is the potential impregnated within us. This part of us is our self-image, our uniqueness, our values and beliefs, our talents, our potential, and our purpose. It is who we really are.

Without this truth—this detergent for your soul—it is impossible to live life in true freedom. When we pursue life as if we were on our own, without God, we soften our potential and give rise to our insecurities. These insecurities are not inherently part of who we are, they are born out of our efforts to earn worth and out of our displaced experiences with disappointment.

The cleanness you are looking for is really a desire for confidence, the innate, unshakable confidence that comes from being yourself. At your core, your unique identity screams to be released. It yearns for you to trust it. It throbs in your soul for you to believe in its beauty. You are not average. You are not unnoticed. Your story is not like anyone else's.

The ultimate cleanse that you can experience is the comprehension that God loves you and that you, by simply being you, are destined to play a beautiful role in the story of the world. Empowered by this knowledge you are free to be true to your authentic self and to trust the person, the quirks, the strengths and weakness that make you the person you are.

Although the world teaches us otherwise, our position determines our condition. Our position is that we are loved and adored by God. We do not and cannot earn God's love because we already have it; we are already positioned as His valued children and therefore the condition of our identity is perfected. Our condition is that we are sinners, and the beautiful thing about God's love for us is that, through Jesus Christ, He cleanses us completely. He is the ultimate detergent for our soul. His grace covers all of our flaws, our mistakes, and our shortcomings; this grace is not earned, it is given freely. Our ability to accept this grace gives us freedom from being in control, because we don't have control over the wondrous grace that has been extended to us, only God does. This grace makes us exactly who we are supposed to be and because of it we don't need to arrive at a new position to be more loved, accepted, or worthy. This position, that of being perfectly loved and perfectly cleansed by God, leads us to a condition of confidence and peace. We have nothing to prove, nothing to earn, and nothing to fear.

Part of the reason we struggle so inherently with insecurity, doubt, fear, and the relentless pressure to prove our worth is because we have been taught the opposite. We learned that our position determines our condition. The better grades we received in school, the smarter we were perceived by others to be. The more successful we were at sports, the more celebrated we were for our athleticism. The higher we climbed in the corporate ladder, the more money we made and more respected we became. The position we achieved— that is, what we were able to earn and do on our own—is the condition of our identity that we perceived to define as our worth.

You are cleansed by God's love and that is enough to claim your position and your condition. You can let go of your efforts to control everything in your life. Take the pressure off and let yourself breathe because God is in control. Because you are a child of God you are perfect in His sight. It is impossible to earn His approval or control your life to be "enough" because you are covered by grace. Moreover, you are loved fiercely by God, and that in and of itself makes you more than enough; it makes you a beloved child of God.

PHYSICAL DETOX
21-Day Cardio Challenge

The position and condition of your life has already been determined and blessed by God. You can, however, take care of the physical condition of your body to ensure that you are honoring it so that you might live long and prosperously. The 21-Day Cardio Challenge is a starter program for someone of any fitness level to facilitate an easy transition into a healthy daily cardiovascular habit of activity.

The purpose of this challenge is to help you create a habit of cardio exercise while you slowly increase your cardiovascular endurance and conditioning at the same time. You have two options: the "relaxed," or beginner, option and the "advanced," or already actively fit, option. The program will walk you through seven three-day sequences, starting with a commitment of just 10 minutes per day and building to a 40-minute workout by day 21. Please keep in mind that this is a program intended not to overwhelm you, so listen to your body as you go and celebrate that you are incorporating a little more movement each day into your life.

The exercise key below explains each exercise as well as the intensity level at which each exercise should be performed. If for any reason you experience pain from an exercise, modify the exercise or substitute it with one that doesn't cause you pain. Both versions of this cardio challenge—the "relaxed" version and the "advanced" version—are presented for you to choose from; select the appropriate challenge by assessing your current fitness level. If you have been actively exercising during the past three to six months, with an average of working out at least three times per week, then the "advanced" version will be a good fit for you. If you haven't been physically active in a while or are recovering from an injury, then the "relaxed" version will be the perfect place for you to start.

RELAXED WORKOUT

10-MINUTE RELAXED WORKOUT (DAYS 1–3)

Duration:	Exercise:
1 Minute	High Knees
1 Minute	Modified Jumping Jacks
2 Minutes	Medium Walking
2 Minutes	Brisk Walking
2 Minutes	Medium Walking
1 Minute	Modified Jumping Jacks
1 Minute	High Knees

15-MINUTE RELAXED WORKOUT (DAYS 4–6)

Duration:	Exercise:
[Repeat 3 Rounds of the Following]:	
1 Minute	Easy Walking
1 Minute	Medium Walking
2 Minutes	Brisk Walking
1 Minute	Medium Walking

20-MINUTE RELAXED WORKOUT (DAYS 7–9)

Duration:	Exercise:
1 Minute	Standing Bicycles
1 Minute	Modified Jumping Jacks
1 Minute	Modified Burpees
2 Minutes	Easy Walking
2 Minutes	Medium Walking
2 Minutes	Brisk Walking
2 Minutes	Very Brisk Walking
2 Minutes	Brisk Walking
2 Minutes	Medium Walking
2 Minutes	Easy Walking
1 Minute	Modified Burpees
1 Minute	Modified Jumping Jacks
1 Minute	Standing Bicycles

25-MINUTE RELAXED WORKOUT (DAYS 10–12)

Duration:	Exercise:
5 Minutes	Bicycle/Burpee/Jumping Jack Mix
[Repeat 2 Rounds of the Following]:	
4 Minutes	Easy Walking

Duration:	Exercise:
3 Minutes	Medium Walking
2 Minutes	Brisk Walking
1 Minute	Light Jog

30-MINUTE RELAXED WORKOUT (DAYS 13–15)

Duration:	Exercise:
5 Minutes	Bicycle/Burpee/Jumping Jack Mix
5 Minutes	Medium Walking
5 Minutes	Brisk Walking
5 Minutes	Medium Walking
5 Minutes	Brisk Walking
5 Minutes	Bicycle/Burpee/Jumping Jack Mix

35-MINUTE RELAXED WORKOUT (DAYS 16–18)

Duration:	Exercise:
5 Minutes	Medium Walking
[Repeat 6 Rounds of the Following]:	
2 Minutes	Light Jog
3 Minutes	Medium Walking

40-MINUTE RELAXED WORKOUT (DAYS 19–21)

Duration:	Exercise:
[Repeat 2 Rounds of the Following]:	
4 Minutes	Medium Walking
1 Minute	Light Jog
3 Minutes	Medium Walking
1 Minute	Light Jog
2 Minutes	Medium Walking
1 Minute	Light Jog
1 Minute	Medium Walking
1 Minute	Light Jog
2 Minutes	Medium Walking
[Repeat 2 Rounds of the Following]:	
2 Minutes	Modified Jumping Jacks
2 Minutes	Modified Burpees
1 Minute	Easy Walking

ADVANCED WORKOUT

10-MINUTE ADVANCED WORKOUT (DAYS 1–3)

Duration:	Exercise:
1 Minute	Jumping Jacks
1 Minute	Mountain Climbers
2 Minutes	Light Jog or Brisk Walk
2 Minutes	Medium Jog
2 Minutes	Light Jog or Brisk Walk
1 Minute	Mountain Climbers
1 Minute	Jumping Jacks

15-MINUTE ADVANCED WORKOUT (DAYS 4–6)

Duration:	Exercise:
[Repeat 3 Rounds of the Following]:	
1 Minute	Light Jog or Brisk Walk
1 Minute	Medium Jog
2 Minutes	Brisk Jog or Run
1 Minute	Medium Jog

20-MINUTE ADVANCED WORKOUT (DAYS 7–9)

Duration:	Exercise:
1 Minute	Mountain Climbers

Duration:	Exercise:
1 Minute	Jumping Jacks
1 Minute	Burpees
2 Minutes	Easy Jog
2 Minutes	Jog
2 Minutes	Brisk Jog
2 Minutes	Run
2 Minutes	Brisk Jog
2 Minutes	Medium Jog
2 Minutes	Easy Jog
1 Minute	Burpees
1 Minute	Jumping Jacks
1 Minute	Mountain Climbers

25-MINUTE ADVANCED WORKOUT (DAYS 10–12)

Duration:	Exercise:
5 Minutes	Burpee/Jumping Jack Mix
[Repeat 2 Rounds of the Following]:	
4 Minutes	Easy Jog
3 Minutes	Medium Jog
2 Minutes	Run
1 Minute	Medium Jog

30-MINUTE ADVANCED WORKOUT (DAYS 13–15)

Duration:	Exercise:
5 Minutes	Burpee/Jumping Jack Mix
5 Minutes	Medium Jog
5 Minutes	Brisk Jog
5 Minutes	Medium Jog
5 Minutes	Brisk Jog
5 Minutes	Burpee/Jumping Jack Mix

35-MINUTE ADVANCED WORKOUT (DAYS 16–18)

Duration:	Exercise:
5 Minutes	Medium Jog
[Repeat 6 Rounds of the Following]:	
2 Minutes	Light Jog
3 Minutes	Brisk Jog

40-MINUTE ADVANCED WORKOUT (DAYS 19–21)

Duration:	Exercise:
[Repeat 2 Rounds of the Following]:	
4 Minutes	Medium Jog
1 Minute	Run
3 Minutes	Medium Jog

Duration:	Exercise:
1 Minute	Run
2 Minutes	Medium Jog
1 Minute	Run
1 Minute	Medium Jog
1 Minute	Run
2 Minutes	Medium Jog
[Repeat 2 Rounds of the Following]:	
2 Minutes	Jumping Jacks
2 Minutes	Burpees
1 Minute	Easy Jog

EXERCISE KEY:

RELAXED EXERCISE KEY/EXPLANATION:

Exercise:	Intensity Effort/Description:
Modified Jumping Jacks	65% effort// Like a jumping jack, but instead of jumping, simply move your legs out on one side—from side to side—so that this stays a low-impact exercise. Move your arms, with your elbows straight, from a relaxed position at your side all the way above your head until your hands clap, and then repeat.

Exercise:	Intensity Effort/Description:
High Knees	65% effort// Standing in place, lift one knee up at a time, as high as you can, and then place it back on the ground, switching legs as you go. This is similar to a high-knee marching movement, however, you are staying in place.
Standing Bicycles	70% effort// In a standing position, maintain a tall posture. Place both hands behind the back of your head with your elbows pointing outward to each side. Lift the left knee from your standing position, and while bending slightly at the waist, move and twist your right elbow down toward the knee to meet the knee. Repeat the movement with the right knee and left elbow, and then continue alternating to complete the exercise.
Modified Burpees	70% effort// Starting from a standing position, bend down into a squatting position, placing your hands on a stable chair. Once your hands are positioned on the chair, step or jump both feet backward so that your body is in a diagonal line from the chair. Pause for a moment, then step or jump your feet back toward the chair and stand up fully. Repeat the exercise and move quickly.

Exercise:	Intensity Effort/Description:
Easy Walking	70% effort// This is a walking pace at which you might leisurely walk a dog.
Medium Walking	80% effort// This is the walking pace you would use when walking in a hurry, but are still able to keep up a leisurely conversation.
Brisk Walking	85% effort// This is the walking pace you would use if you were in a hurry to get out of the rain.
Very Brisk Walking	90% effort// This is your best variation of speed walking and is the fastest you can walk.
Light Jog	95% effort// This is slightly faster than your very brisk walking pace and is a light jog where you will use your arms to guide your body into a movement pattern that mimics running.

ADVANCED EXERCISE KEY/EXPLANATION:

Exercise:	Intensity Effort / Description:
Jumping Jacks	60% effort// Perform a basic jumping jack, making sure your feet leave the ground and your arms come all the way above your head, with your hands clapping together at the top to complete each repetition.

Exercise:	Intensity Effort / Description:
Mountain Climbers	75% effort// From a plank, or push-up position, keep your arms extended in a 90-degree angle from the ground, tighten your abdominals, and bring one knee at a time upward toward your belly button, switching your legs quickly as if your legs were running, or doing a lateral high-knee movement from the plank position.
Burpees	70% effort// Starting from a standing position, squat and then drop your hands to the floor, jumping your feet out to land in a plank, or push-up position. From the plank position, perform a push-up and then jump your feet back so that you are in a forward fold, squat position. From that forward fold, squat position jump upward, with your arms over your head, as high as you can, making sure your feet leave the ground. Land your jump, ending in the standing position, and repeat.
Easy Jogging	70% effort// This is a light run or jogging pace at which you are barely exerting yourself and you are able to have an extensive conversation while you do it. You should feel like you could do this pace for miles.

Exercise:	Intensity Effort / Description:
Medium Jogging	80% effort// This is your "basic" jogging pace and is one at which you feel good but that you wouldn't want to hold an extensive conversation while doing it.
Brisk Jogging	85% effort// This is a "tempo" pace, meaning it is a pace that you push yourself but don't overexert yourself; it is a pushed pace that is sustainable.
Run	90% effort// This is above a tempo pace, but not a sprint.
Hard Run	95% effort// This is equivalent to a sprint or your fastest running pace.

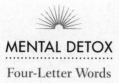

MENTAL DETOX
Four-Letter Words

We all know the list of "four-letter words" to avoid using. They are the words that are crass, vulgar, rude, mean, and, well, just bad words. Similarly, there are some "four-letter words" that you need to eliminate from your internal vocabulary, which will help clean the current condition of your mind. These words might not be limited to four letters, in fact, they might be longer words, critical adjectives, or even phrases about yourself that run in your mind. They are words that need to be removed from your life. Take three minutes and come up with the five most pervasive "four-letter words" that you have called yourself in your past. Write them down and then rewrite them in a positive light.

"Four-Letter Words"/Negative Self-Phrases:

1) ....

2) ....

3) ....

4) ....

5) ....

"Four-Letter Words"/New Phrases:

1) ....

2) ....

3) ....

4) ....

5) ....

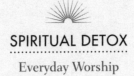

SPIRITUAL DETOX
Everyday Worship

O Lord, I will honor and praise your name, for you are my God.
You do such wonderful things! You planned them long ago,
and now you have accomplished them. (Isaiah 25:1)

The most effective way to cleanse your soul on a daily basis is to submit yourself to a lifestyle of worship. Worship comes in all sizes, shapes, and varieties. It is whatever you do that makes your soul sing. Live your life in such a way that the way you live glorifies God. You can worship through the small interactions you have with others, through the thoughts you choose, through small acts of kindness and service toward others and through engaging in the joy of life by living in the present moment. Everyday worship is an attitude. It is the attitude that life is beautiful and that God is good. Equipped with that attitude, your life will become a living and breathing testimony of worship. You will find that your attitude doesn't just uplift others and honor God, but it will uplift you as well. Worship is the detergent for our hearts that we might live consistently with an attitude of gratitude; such an attitude allows us to live according to the words of Psalm 51:10, with a "clean heart" and "renewed spirit."

....

Father, teach me how to relinquish my desire for
control. Create in me a clean heart and a clean
attitude that I might know just how deeply I
am loved. In the loving name of Jesus, Amen.

THE ORDINARY

The Truth: You have greatness within you.

*There is greatness within you, and it is up to you to step up
and take on the challenge of living life to the fullest.*

American Gladiators Greatness

I don't know if you remember the '90s show *American Gladiators*. Unlike stories about superheroes, *American Gladiators*
was a real-time game show with real everyman competitors
and larger-than-life gladiators. The show capitalized on a
David-and-Goliath theme, where the real heroes weren't the
gladiators, but rather the underdogs who stepped up to take a
challenge that seemed larger than life.

My brother Nick and I would high-five each other every
time a contestant overtook a gladiator. We thought that if
someone as normal-looking as a contestant could triumph
over seemingly impossible circumstances, then, even just as
kids, we could do the same thing. The *American Gladiators*

contestants were our first exposure to the belief system that an underdog can really win.

In 2007, NBC decided to revive the *American Gladiators* show, wanting to celebrate everyday, true American heroes. Fondly recalling my childhood memories of how much the show encouraged my spirit, I decided to try out at the open calling.

I showed up at the Chicago auditions to a line that wrapped around the warehouse feeling shy, intimidated, and unqualified. Hundreds of fitness professionals waited hours for the chance to try out. Reluctantly, I stayed in line, feeling extremely out of place and nowhere close to being good enough.

After hours of waiting in line, I made it to the front. The audition consisted of an obstacle course race, a pull-up challenge, a sprint, and then an immediate on-camera interview with the show's producers from NBC. I sweated the pull-ups because I saw a girl before me knock out seventeen like it was nothing. She probably could have done one-arm pull-ups if she had wanted. I was way out of my league. I hated pull-ups and I certainly couldn't do more than a few at my very best effort.

Finally, when my turn came I did my best and felt decent about my audition. I managed about five pull-ups, way below the average for those auditioning, but I did excel at the speed and agility challenges that were part of the obstacle course. After I completed my final wind sprint I was still out of breath when I was seated at a foldout table in front of three cameras and three NBC producers. I was asked a series of rapid-fire questions and then shuffled out the door.

A few days went by and I didn't hear anything.

Then almost a week later, the phone rang.

I was one of ten selected for round one of callbacks. I progressed past round one and was invited to round two, a private hour-long on-camera interview with three producers. It went well, but I was still plagued with nerves and doubt because I so wanted to live out my childhood dream and was worried that I wasn't going to be "good enough" to be selected.

A few days later the executive producer called and asked me to pack my bags to fly to Los Angeles the next day. They wanted me on the show.

Unfortunately I never made it to L.A. I had literally just been promoted at my job—the same day I got the call from NBC. If I went, I would lose my promotion and the job, so I stayed. Even though I turned down my opportunity to compete on *American Gladiators,* the experience gained me immeasurably more than any cash prize I could have won by being on the show.

The prize I won was a newfound belief in my potential. Who knew I had hero potential within me? I certainly didn't. But it was there. It is there for you, too. Just as the NBC producers saw within me a potential to be a great underdog that I couldn't see, so, too, is there a potential in you that you aren't currently acknowledging.

So many of us are drawn toward heroes because heroes represent the potential we all suspect is hidden within us. Heroes are the epitome of greatness, for they are ordinary people who do extraordinary things with their lives. This translation of the ordinary into the extraordinary awakens within us a hope that we, too, might be able to unleash our own inner greatness to do great things that seem beyond what we might ordinarily be able to do.

The trouble is that we never see ourselves for who we really are. Even though we are the main characters in our own story, we are usually the last to see what our life actually means. We sell ourselves short, limiting our potential and putting boundaries on the story our lives will tell. Somewhere along the way we stopped believing we were extraordinary and instead settled for being just ordinary. We forgot what should never be forgotten: we are called to do extraordinary things. In order to do extraordinary things, though, we must be willing to offer our ordinary gifts to God, and we do that by taking action on the life that has been laid out before us. God awakens the hero within us by taking our best and making it better because with Him on our side, we are unstoppable.

We are not called to live boring, ordinary, or average lives. We are called to be heroes. Ordinary people who do extraordinary things because of God's love.

PHYSICAL DETOX
Gallon Challenge

Any gladiators out there already know this, but there is a magic that is found in water. One small change to your diet in this arena will grant you almost instant results. The magic is that water is metabolically revving your body.

The natural simplicity of water often gets overlooked but it is a lodestone for your health. Most people are chronically dehydrated. Dehydration not only retards our metabolism, but it also affects our energy levels and our body's internal ability to rid itself of toxins. Additionally, there is no better skin product than water. The effects of a well-hydrated body outperform any beauty product on the market. Moreover, for the purposes of this cleanse, water is the ultimate internal cleanse for your body. It flushes out your organs, your digestive system, your muscles, and your skin.

Set yourself up for success by starting the day (yes, even before your cup of coffee), with at least 16 ounces of ice-cold water.

Your detox today is to take on "The Gallon Challenge." The gallon challenge is simple: drink one gallon, 128 ounces, of water per day for the next seven days. Below are some recommendations to help make this detox step successful:

- Tally your ounces as you go to keep track. Figure out exactly how many bottles of water you need to drink per day and then use a Sharpie to mark on the bottle each time you have finished a bottle. Fill the bottle up and start over.
- Always have a water bottle with you—in your car or in your purse.
- Be ready to pee more frequently—it's a good sign that your body is ridding itself of toxins.
- Match your water intake to any additional caffeine you take in—for example, if you drink a 12-ounce cup of coffee, chase it with 12 ounces of water before you even think about pouring your next cup of coffee.

I recommend using one plastic bottle for the day. Keep a Sharpie in your purse and add a mark to the bottle once you drink it and refill it. This will allow you to stay on track with exactly how many ounces you have had for the day. Even better, take the challenge with a friend; this will encourage you to increase the tally marks and give it the competitive nature of a game.

MENTAL DETOX
Rewriting Your Potential

Rewriting the words in your mind is like breaking any habit. Habits are best broken by substitution, not removal. Those who really create new, positive habits in their lives are those who take the symptoms of their bad habits and rewrite them into new, positive behaviors.

To rewrite your thoughts you need to properly prep the mind for substitution.

Today I want you to rewrite your potential. Literally. Pick which of the phrases below most resonates with you, or make up your own phrase, and then take some paper and handwrite the phrase twenty times. Twenty times may seem excessive, but it is the number of repetitions recommended by most psychologists for memorization or internalization of a phrase.

"I can do anything."
"I have great potential within me."
"I am strong, I am smart, I am special."
"I believe in myself."
*"I am who God created me to be and that is all I need
    to be."*

"God put greatness into me, I will trust Him and honor who He made me to be."

"Each day, in every way, I am becoming better and better."

SPIRITUAL DETOX

Got it Good

And I am certain that God, who began the good work within you, will continue his work until it is finished on the day when Christ Jesus returns. (Philippians 1:6)

You've got it good. God has breathed potential and greatness into you. Having it "good"—and celebrating it with a "got it good" list—means that you are blessed extensively in the small, daily details of life. To be included on a "got it good" list are friends, family, children, the provision of a job, the community where you live, your church, the beauty of nature that you can enjoy, happiness, holidays, pets, adventure, fruits of the spirit, and opportunities to learn and grow, just to name a few examples.

You are His child, handcrafted and purposed by Him to live. The most exciting thing about this potential is that God will carry it to completion in you. Your spiritual detox is to consider the innate talents and abilities God has sown into you as well as the gifts He has interwoven into your life. They are often so intricately woven into us that we take them for granted. Create a "got it good" list of these talents and keep it with you throughout the day. Add to it every time you think of something about yourself or your life that is worthy of celebration. Remember to acknowledge the gifts, talents, and personality traits that make you good at being you.

....

Father, I believe that You have destined me
for greatness and that You have more than an
ordinary life planned for me. Help me fight my
fears of averageness and of the ordinary and
teach me to fix my eyes on the extraordinary
details of the beautiful life You have given
me. In the great name of Jesus, Amen.

Got It Good List

1) ....

2) ....

3) ....

4) ....

5) ....

LIMITED THINKING

The Truth: God makes all things possible in our lives.

God plus anything makes it better, particularly when that "anything" is you.

Divine Mathematics

I'm embarrassed to admit that I need to brush up on my multiplication tables. Math was never my forte, but I did always manage to get good grades in the subject. As with all subjects that I didn't like, I mastered the art of short-term memorization to get by successfully. Secretly, I am actually looking forward to when my daughter Ellie starts school so that I am forced back into relearning some of the basics as I help her with her homework.

One type of math I have learned to be good at, though, is God's math. I was a slow learner to start, but over time I have come to embrace the presence of the divine mathematics that reigns in my life. The beautiful thing about God's math is that I'm barely involved at all, which is perhaps why I can claim to be good at it. God's math is something that the only participation required of us is to believe in it. That's our entire role: be-lieving in and trusting in the Master calculator.

God covers the basics of mathematics with precision in His reign over our lives. God plus anything is infinitely im-proved; He has addition perfected. He is the Master of sub-traction; He can subtract anything from our life that hinders us, harms us, or holds us back. Because of Him, we are di-vided from the world and set apart for glory. His division makes us special and equips us to love others as His represen-tatives. And finally, He is the King of multiplication. When God multiplies, He uses joy. He magnifies the glories of the Heavens in our lives through the great overflow of His love onto us.

Traditional mathematics is based on linear thinking and logical progressions. It is a system that depends on patterns, absolutes, and quantifiable logic. Divine mathematics is dif-ferent. It exists outside of logic, beyond the linear trajectory and is unpredictable. The only thing predictable about God's math is that it has power to change our lives in magnificent ways.

Too often we limit our lives by confining ourselves to lin-ear, human thinking. We see ourselves with human eyes and as such we limit the potential of our lives based on the limita-tions of our own minds. God sees us in ways we could never see ourselves. God's math is not like ours.

God plus anything makes it better, particularly when that "any-thing" is you.

God plus you equals courage.
God plus you equals confidence.

> God plus you equals legacy.
> God plus you equals freedom.
> God plus you equals happiness.
> God plus you equals certainty.
> God plus you equals authenticity.

God wants a relationship with us; He wants to pair up with us and be by our side. And since He gave us free will, He cannot force the relationship—it must come from our own volition. When we invite Him into our lives, He adds to us more than we could have possibly imagined or asked for.

I spent years of my life trying to remove negative things—addictions, toxic thoughts, sinful patterns—from my life on my own, but as it turns out, there are certain things in my life that I can't subtract out myself. I can't do it, but God, the Master Subtractor, can.

God can subtract anything from our lives that holds us back or hinders us.

> God subtracts our insecurities.
> God subtracts our fears.
> God subtracts our limitations.
> God subtracts our doubts.
> God subtracts our sin.
> God subtracts our selfishness.

One of the most foundational yearnings put onto the heart of every human being is a desire to do something that matters. All you have to do is watch the way we celebrate celebrities and elevate the famous to see that we have put value on standing out. We all want to know that we are special. We all want to know that we matter. And, most of all, we all want to know that our lives mean something. God divides us from the world and sets us aside with purpose . . . that we might be a light of His love to others . . . and it is this Divine division that gives us confidence in our purpose.

God divides us from the world for a reason.

> God divides us by setting us apart as special.
> God divides us away from negative and toxic cir-
> cumstances.
> God divides us, making us stand out as a beacon of
> light to others.
> God divides us from our sinful ways.
> God divides us from mediocrity by gifting us with
> talent and potential.

I think the addition, subtraction, and division skills of God are amazing, but when it comes to the way He uses the power of multiplication, I believe He shows off. It is in His multiplication of my life that I am most humbled and in awe, because it is a result of His multiplication that my life over-flows with joy, favor, and blessings. Multiplication is God's way of taking our little and making it much.

God multiplies blessings and magnifies His favor in our lives by pouring out His love on us.

> God multiplies favor.
> God multiplies our joy.
> God multiplies provisions.

God multiplies our love.
God multiplies our creativity.
God multiplies our opportunities.
God multiplies our impact.
God multiplies our voice.

We can relearn the mathematics of life if we simply open our minds to see that God's math is different from ours. God takes His relationship with us seriously—it is precious to Him—and He uses addition, subtraction, division, and multiplication to magnify our lives in ways that will bless us and help us grow closer to Him. The closer we are to Him, the greater our reflection of His love out to the world will be, and that is the greatest outcome of all. With God's math, anything and everything is possible.

PHYSICAL DETOX
Twenty and Thirty

Two simple numbers to keep in mind as you start each day are: twenty and thirty. One secret of those who have a high-performing and calorie-burning metabolism is that they eat breakfast every morning. More than simply eating breakfast, eating breakfast within the first thirty minutes of waking up can have a significant impact on your metabolic stimulus. Additionally, by including at least 20 grams of protein in what you choose for breakfast, you will set your metabolism up for optimal performance throughout the day. So, remember: focus on getting your 20 grams of protein within thirty minutes after waking for optimal body function and fat burning.

To help you implement your new habit of "twenty and thirty," here are some options for breakfasts that boast at least 20 grams of protein: whey protein shake made with almond milk, baked egg white muffins or hard-boiled egg whites (5 egg whites), Greek yogurt with a scoop of whey protein mixed in, Ezekiel bread with protein-packed natural peanut or almond butter with a glass of milk or almond milk.

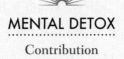

MENTAL DETOX
Contribution

We all want to know that our lives make a contribution to this world and to those around us. God takes what we contribute to ourselves and toward others and multiplies its effect. Therefore, the better we know ourselves, the more of ourselves we can give, and the larger contribution we can make. When you know what you love to do, know how God has gifted you with talents and passions, and know that you want to help others, then you can really make a contribution in this world.

Use the following equations to assess how you might be able to contribute with your talents, skills, and voice to the world around you:

Contribution = ((Personal Interest) + (Personal Gift) + (Personal Passion)) x [Heart]

Below is the math in my personal example of completing the contribution equation:

Trish's Contribution = ((Words/Writing/Speaking) [+] (Outgoing Personality/Talkative/Self-Reflective Nature) [+] (Passion to Help Others Break Out of Self-Imposed Bondage and Self-Doubt)) [x] (Desire to Really Make a Difference in the World and to be a Reflection of God's Love)

In shorter terms for my example:

((Books) [+] (Self-Reflection) [+] (You)) [x] (God) [=] Contribution/Impact

Now, fill out your own contribution equation in the blank equation provided below:

Contribution = ((Personal Interest) [+] (Personal Gift) [+] (Personal Passion)) [x] [Heart]

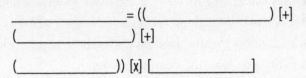

_____ = ((_____) [+]
(_____) [+]
(_____)) [x] [_____]

SPIRITUAL DETOX
Generating Generosity

Give, and you will receive. Your gift will return to you in full—pressed down, shaken together to make room for more, running over, and poured into your lap. The amount you give will determine the amount you get back. (Luke 6:38)

Generosity is one of the character attributes that God multiplies in us once we choose to express it ourselves. The more generous we are, the more God gives us and entrusts to us to be generous with. By being generous—with our love, our time, our money, our talents, and our words—God multiplies our resources.

The act of generosity has a trickle-down effect that works like a ripple effect. The more we give, the more we have to give. It's a small example of God's multiplication and how He can multiply the small gifts we give and make them into larger contributions to others. So never underestimate small acts of generosity. It doesn't matter how much you have to give, what matters is that you have the heart of a giver.

Think about the people who have most touched your life by their generosity; identify at least three people. Contact at least one of them this week to compliment them on their generosity and to thank them for the positive example they have set for you to emulate. As you consider the example of these people in your life, and the positive impact they have had upon you, pray for a deepened spirit of generosity that you might become more like them. Pray that God will multiply your heart and generate blessings through you by what you are able to give to others.

....

Father, forgive me for my limited, small thinking.
I believe that through You all things are possible.
Show me how to live out that truth in my mind
that I might have the courage to follow the big
dreams You have put on my heart. Create in
me a spirit of generosity. In the name of Jesus,
through whom all things are possible, Amen.

UNTAPPED POTENTIAL

*The Truth: God has breathed into
you potential and purpose.*

*God created you with incredible potential; your job is to discover and
live out that potential by being the best version of yourself.*

Wolfram Alpha

When I was a kid I loved looking into the sky and placing my best guess on where an airplane was headed. It was the type of game that allowed me to daydream. The thought of hundreds of passengers flying through the air above toward an unknown destination was so romantic, so outlandish, and so big that my little brain had trouble imagining it.

The day I found out about Wolfram Alpha is the day I realized just how much I didn't know about what I really have available to me. Wolfram Alpha is a technological capability built into Siri on the iOS platform. When you ask Siri about the airplanes above you at that given moment, within seconds she provides a detailed report of what aircrafts are currently miles above your head.

As I write this JetBlue Airways flight 891 is 34,000 feet above me, Republic Airlines flight 3436 is 14,700 feet above me, and Atlantic Southeast Airlines flight 6004 is 10,000 feet high. But the information isn't just limited to that. I hold in my hand the type of carrier that is flying, the angle of their trajectory, and the slant distance they are in approximation to me. I can type the flight numbers into Google and find out exactly where the plane originated and where its final destination will be. Gone is my childhood guessing game.

Wolfram Alpha is a mostly untapped technology within Siri. You probably sort of know what to do with Siri, but you might not have a good grasp on the true potential of its functionality.

The promise of potential is simply captivating. It sings to us of hope and of something beyond what we can currently see. Our potential is a gift from God, breathed into us at our birth. Like any gift, potential doesn't unwrap itself; we must be the ones to unwrap it. We have to choose to open it up.

Most of us know that we have a gift within us, but we hesitate to open it. We get stuck in identities handed to us in high school or in the expectations of our parents. We listen to our own internal tapes of things people have said about us and allow those words to define who we think we are. Sometimes we don't even see ourselves at all—instead we feel numb, average, and forgettable and we fool those around us into thinking that we know ourselves, even though we feel lost. Regardless of the reason why we don't untie the ribbons of our potential, one thing holds true: we all have more to us than we know.

I believe we live our lives according to the characteristics of identity that we believe ourselves to have. In other words, we either liberate or limit ourselves and our potential by what we choose to believe is possible. What we think about ourselves is what we become.

To tap into our potential, we must be ourselves. Not being oneself is like having an iPhone and only using it as a phone. Locked within us are amazing talents, like Wolfram Alpha, just waiting to be explored.

Too often we attempt to forge our own identities within the confines of our own limited imaginations. As a result, we minimize our potential and we short-sell our purpose. We don't need to understand or be able to see everything about ourselves in order to journey along our path, in the same way the passengers on JetBlue flight 891 trust the pilots to direct them to their correct destination.

You have a Creator, and He put something great within you. Open your gift and share it with those around you. You may not yet know how to use your Wolfram Alpha technology, but trust in God and continue to practice using your gift.

PHYSICAL DETOX
Shopping Rewrite

You can maximize what your body can achieve by cleaning up your shopping list. Initially, the adjustment to buying more fresh food and fewer processed goods may seem more expensive, but consider the difference in your grocery bill as an investment in your health future. When shopping at the grocery store, always shop the perimeter of the store first, as you should be able to get 90 percent of your cart filled with "clean," whole foods. Reserve aisle shopping for the final 10 percent of odds and ends that you might need. If you do need to buy anything that is prepackaged, manufactured, or premade, make an effort to read the nutrition and ingredient label and try to keep the total number of ingredients for any product under five. If the ingredients include words that you can't pronounce, it's probably best that item doesn't end up in your shopping cart and ultimately your stomach.

What comes into your house is up to you. It is imperative to always shop with a list so as to not get distracted by nonessentials or packaged foods that are on sale.

To download your own copy of my Clean Eating Grocery Shopping Checklist, go to www.trishblackwell.com/cleanshoppinglist.

MENTAL DETOX
Original Thoughts

Tapping into your potential and your dreams can become more natural for you by engaging your mind creatively. This exercise will give your mind permission to flow freely, ultimately training your mind to be less inhibited. As you begin to think more freely you will start seeing yourself with more possibilities than ever before. This exercise is simple: you are going to string words together into a sentence that no one has ever thought of before. Get crazy with this and let your creativity shine.

As a guideline, fill in the following two MabLibs to get

yourself started and then give yourself five minutes to allow for "free flow" writing and sentence creation. Your sentences don't need to make sense, just let them be creative and original.

(Pronoun) .... loves (hobby) .... so very much that (pronoun) .... (verb) .... to the (noun) .... and (verb) .... (noun) ....

I always (verb) .... loudly and (verb) .... that (pronoun) .... is the (adjective) .... (noun) .... that exists in the (noun) ....

SPIRITUAL DETOX

Loving More

Dear friends, let us continue to love one another, for love comes from God. Anyone who loves is a child of God and knows God. (1 John 4:7)

Love is the most undertapped resource in us all. Though we talk and think about love a lot, we can all love more.

The crucial component to loving more is to first love ourselves. Many of our own personal insecurities often stem from us not loving ourselves enough. We berate ourselves over small mistakes, we pressure ourselves to try to "do it all," and we often run on a hamster wheel of constant self-criticism.

You *can* learn to love yourself, even if you aren't sure where to start. You cannot give out what you do not first have, which is why it is imperative for you to love yourself first so that you can more authentically love others. List three things that you know you need to celebrate about yourself with more warmth and openness. This exercise will help you see yourself with kindness and celebration, which ultimately will empower you to see the same in others to a degree that you never thought possible before.

My body:
1) ....
2) ....
3) ....

My personality:
1) ....
2) ....
3) ....

My quirks and interests:
1) ....
2) ....
3) ....

....

*Father, I trust Your plan. I trust how You created
me and the potential You placed inside of me.
I believe that You created me with purpose and
for a purpose. I pray that You teach me how to
live out Your calling for my life with confidence.
In the powerful name of Jesus, Amen.*

SELF-DOUBT

The Truth: You are remarkable and special.

*Borrow God's eyes to look past your self-doubt and insecurity
to see the remarkable person God created you to be.*

Unremarkably Different

I can recall the very first time I felt out of place. I was nine
years old and playing on the monkey bars at our local YMCA
with my older brother and his friends, one of whom I had a
crush on. He was redheaded with freckles and he was a fast
swimmer—to a nine-year-old girl, he had it all. Hanging from
my knees, my shirt went over my head and an outburst of
laughter ensued. The laughing turned to teasing and I was
told that I looked like a boy. Pointing to my flat chest they
joked that I would never have a boyfriend and that no one
would ever have a crush on me. My dreams of being a princess
were pierced. Gutted, I fell to the ground to pull my shirt back
down into place. I had never felt more out of place in my life.

Their words and that scene planted the first seeds of insecurity in my heart. As I dwelt on the pain of feeling rejected and unlovely, the hurt intensified. For years as I waited for puberty, I feared that I would never really become a woman, that a boy would never like me, and that I would never be truly beautiful.

Growing up is difficult in different ways for everyone. We are all desperate to fit in—to be accepted by others—and yet paradoxically, we yearn to stand out and be noticed for being special. I wanted to be special, and since I had believed the lie that I wasn't beautiful I threw myself with ferocity into my athletics. I wanted to be out of place—to be special—but to be in place—part of the group—as well.

My master plan didn't work, though. I learned quickly that by standing out too much, or in my case, being highly successful at my sport, I was then excluded for being *too* successful. No matter what I did, I didn't fit in. I couldn't find my place.

My sophomore year at boarding school, everything changed for me. Feeling unlovely, I thought the answer to beauty was found in being skinnier. An anorexic friend offered me a way out. She took me into the stall in our dorm bathroom and taught me how to throw up. She handed me diet pills and she told me which foods never to eat. She was popular, pretty, and rich, so I did everything she said. That day my actions (and subsequent eating disorder) taught my mind to believe that my body would never be good enough.

In some ways I felt like God had let me down. I was mad that He hadn't given me the body I wanted and I hated how my mind was consumed by constant negativity. I wondered if God had made a mistake when He made me.

Our feelings of insecurity and self-doubt are birthed early in life, and we often feel unnoticeable and unremarkable. Secretly, we just want to fit in, yet conversely, we also want to stand out and be special. This conflict spirals us into a state of confused identity and makes us all too familiar with always feeling a little bit out of place, or unremarkably different. We *are,* however, remarkable and we *are* different from any other human being that has ever existed on this planet. It is in our difference that lays our greatest beauty; unfortunately, for many of us it takes years to realize that being out of place is exactly what gives us our place.

There are so many ways "not _____ enough" finds its way as insecurity into our perceived identities. For me, these are some of the ones that like to creep into my mind:

Not *skinny* enough . . .
Not *smart* enough . . .
Not *tall* enough . . .
Not *successful* enough . . .
Not *pretty* enough . . .
Not *funny* enough . . .
Not *outgoing* enough . . .

There are thousands of possibilities in this "enough" equation that leaves so many of us feeling underwhelmed with ourselves and overwhelmed with life. Whatever your "not _____ enough" is, the source of this insecurity is the same as mine: fear.

We fear, which expresses itself through self-doubt, self-comparison, and self-limiting thoughts, because we know not who we really are. We fear because ultimately we are afraid that we aren't wonderfully made. We fear because we are afraid that we don't matter. Whenever fear is given the loudest voice it creates a "not enough" mindset, which then distorts reality like a funhouse mirror. The problem is that we are using our own limited eyesight when we should be seeing ourselves through God's eyes. Using God's eyes to view yourself removes the distortion.

God sees you as wonderfully made. He doesn't see the flaws that you see—His eyes are filled with mercy, love, and grace. He sees who you are, who you will be, and who you *can* be. It is up to us to close the difference between those states of being. Borrow God's eyes to see yourself. Use them to re-visit those painful memories. Use them on your hope for tomorrow. Through God's eyes your perceived flaws disappear and you will quickly find the place God has prepared for you to be.

PHYSICAL DETOX
Daily Success Setup

One very easy way to live a remarkable life is to set yourself up with remarkable daily habits. Set yourself up for success each and every day by starting your mornings with a *Daily Success Setup,* or DSS routine. Your DSS routine should include at least three small tasks, but no more than five, and it should demand less than five total minutes of time from your schedule. It is essentially a list of daily routines that help make your life work best for you when they are performed. By performing your DSS at the beginning of each day you simultaneously prepare your mind to continue along a pathway of success. Completing the DSS communicates to your subconscious that you have already started the day with enthusiasm and success, and it leaves you with confidence and the innate desire to continue that pattern.

Your DSS should be simple. It could include some of the following suggestions:

- Making your bed
- Stretching your body for two minutes
- Taking five deep, slow breaths
- Writing briefly in a gratitude journal
- Getting on your knees for a minute of prayer
- Doing a minute of abdominal work or a plank hold
- Smiling at yourself in the mirror for 30 seconds
- Packing your lunch for the day
- Calling someone you love and wishing them a good day
- Writing out your top three goals and priorities for the day

Not only will your DSS list help motivate you to continue successfully tackling tasks that arise throughout your day, but it will strengthen your psyche to think confidently about the day ahead and the challenges that will inevitably test your mind. Use the space below to write out five habits that you are willing to commit to your DSS list. Be intentional for the next three days about completing your DSS habits in the morning before the rest of your day starts.

....

....

....

....

....

MENTAL DETOX
Body Type Acceptance

Feeling insecure about your body can make you feel out of place everywhere you go because you feel out of place in the skin you're in. There is no such thing as a perfect body. Every body is beautiful in its own way, though unfortunately we live in a world that inundates our expectations with standards of unrealistic images of what beauty is. This Photoshopped standard of manufactured beauty tells us that we aren't good enough unless we strive to achieve a media-produced, flawless image . . . an ideal body that doesn't actually exist. There are armies of people who put together these manufactured images, but since what they do is behind the scenes, we end up believing the façade that such "perfect" beauty actually exists when in fact it doesn't.

Your body type is unchangeable. It is part of your genetic makeup. Your mental detox for body type acceptance starts with embracing the truth that the body type you were given at birth *is* beautiful. More often than not we live life thinking that the grass is greener on the other side of the fence; in the case of our bodies we waste countless amounts of emotional energy wishing away the body type that we have in lieu of one that we covet in someone else. The sneaky secret about body types is that every body type sees something in the other body types that they like better than what they have in theirs.

There are three main body types: ectomorphs, meso-morphs, and endomorphs. Ectomorphs have a natural ten-dency to be long and lean, mesomorphs have a more muscular and athletic build, and endomorphs are prone to weight gain and body-fat storage. Typically, you have primarily one type as your dominant structure and then a secondary type as your subdominant body type. For example, a naturally athletic per-son who has the propensity to easily gain weight would be considered primarily as a mesomorph with an endomorphic secondary nature. A similar athlete with a leaner build would be considered a mesomorph with ectomorphic tendencies.

In addition to the basic biological body types, our bodies have natural shapes that cannot be changed. A triangle, an in-verted triangle, a rectangle, a thin rectangle, an oval, and an hourglass are some of the physical shapes our bodies naturally take on. In such cases, some people store extra weight and body fat in their lower body, some in their upper body, and some in the middle of their body, all according to their natural body shape.

Embrace the body type that God has given you by first identifying what body type you have. Next, assess yourself as a whole and determine which shape your body naturally tends toward. Once you have assessed both types, you can start ac-cepting your body for how it is. Accept the fact that your body type is unchangeable. Doing so will release you into a place of freedom to accept what you've got because it's what you'll always have. The grass always seems greener on the other side of the fence, not because it is, but because we can't see the poop in the other yard. Water your own grass by treating your body with kindness, appreciation, and respect and your grass will be the greenest of greens.

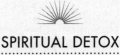

SPIRITUAL DETOX
Godly Conversations

The Lord is close to all who call on him, yes, to all who call on him in truth. (Psalm 145:18)

One of the most effective ways to transform your thought life from being unremarkable to being extraordinary is by improving your prayer life. Prayer saturates and surrounds your soul with a spiritual perspective that will also guard your mind. It is with guarded minds that we can consciously choose to cling to the truth and to reject the lies—the "not enoughs"—in our lives.

Prayer is simply a conversation with God, how we develop a friendship with Him. There is no wrong way to pray.

One of my favorite ways to connect with family and friends is to share my daily *haut/bas* (pronounced "ooooh/bahh"). Translated from French, *haut/bas* means "high"/"low"; by sharing the highest or best part of my day and the lowest or worst part of my day with those I love, I feel more connected.

To inspire you to have more Godly conversations through-out your days consider sharing your *haut/bas* with Him at the end of the day or simply as you progress through your day. God cares about the little things like your *haut/bas*. He cares about your heart and He cares about your day.

....

Father, detox my mind from the self-doubts that linger in its shadows. Help me really understand that I am special and created uniquely by You, the Master Craftsman. Deepen my daily desire to connect with You, let our quiet times together become foundational to my life. In the remarkable name of Jesus, Amen.

BUSYNESS

The Truth: Solitude is a way to grow in confidence.

The still moments of life give us the most opportunity to grow, when we can learn to step outside of the busyness of life and simply be in the present.

14,000 Hours Under Water

As a competitive swimmer I spent more than 14,000 hours underwater in my career. Swimming is a sport where silence reigns. The quiet that came with swimming became my daily self-reflection time. For many years, I trained up to four hours per day in the water. That's a lot of time to have your head submerged; it's a lot of time to be alone with your own thoughts. The pool became my think tank, my therapist. It forced me, someone who loves the distraction of being around others, to be alone.

Spending time alone is a foundational practice that carves out space in our minds to see ourselves for who we are. This alone time isn't a luxury; rather, it is a necessity. Being alone permits us to explore ourselves and to discover the intricacies of our identities, which in turn equip us to combat insecurity when it arises. In order to be confident, we need to know who we are and need to be able to be alone with ourselves and with our thoughts. Alone time is not only crucial to self-discovery, but it is also an important component to claiming confidence in our lives.

We live in a world where it is difficult to be alone. Our lives are filled with static and distraction, both of which ultimately deter us from our destiny. Even in the moments we find ourselves physically alone, the constant connectedness of social media surrounds us with thousands. One of the most effective ways to liberate oneself from old patterns of insecure thinking is to spend time alone in self-reflection. This type of solitude is essential to uncluttering the mind. It is the clutter in our minds that causes many of our insecurities. Spending time alone, particularly in quiet silence, opens our hearts to hear the whispers of God. It silences the shouting of the world and brings us to a place we belong.

There is no right or wrong way to incorporate more still-ness in your life, but you must do it. The quiet time you allow yourself is a powerful tool that will help you detox the doubts that so often become insecurities in your mind.

What gets scheduled gets done. As an athlete—as a swim-mer in my past and now as an endurance runner and triathlete—my solitude is scheduled alongside my workouts. The good news is that you don't have to spend 14,000 hours with your head underwater or put in ten miles on the tread-mill to successfully incorporate solitude into your life. Just make it a priority and schedule it, whether it is by attaching it to a workout, a walk, or just to an afternoon pause on your front porch swing. This solitude is essential to uncluttering the mind and understanding our identity. It is in knowing our identity and owning it with confidence that we can most effectively combat the attacks of insecurity that come against us. It's difficult to believe the lies insecurity tempts you with when you know firmly who you are; and to know who you are you must step away from the hustle and bustle of life and step into the stillness of solitude.

As we learn through the stillness to embrace how God created us to be we will learn to shed the shackles of insecurity that keep us from living life to the fullest. Embrace more stillness in your daily routine and you will experience more mental and emotional space for your confidence to grow. Whatever you do, find a way to get some time alone, even if you have to stick your head underwater to do it.

PHYSICAL DETOX
Scheduling Solitude

Alone time can be done in a variety of ways and doesn't have to be the same every day. Create a habit of intentionally incorporating alone time into your lifestyle and try to stick to a scheduled time for yourself, throwing in new things for variety as needed. Below are a few examples to inspire you:

- 15 minutes of "quiet time" first thing in the morning. Quiet time can be a time to meditate, read, stretch, or simply be free of distraction and *noise*.

- Go for a run or walk without music.
- Eat lunch or dinner at a restaurant by yourself.
- Take a weekend trip with no itinerary.
- Gratitude journaling.
- Drive somewhere new and create your own adventure.
- Write (or type) out your prayers as a form of journaling.
- Leave your smartphone in another room when you have your cup of coffee.
- Turn the TV off at night, as well as your phone, for an hour to read or take a bath.
- Schedule a "me" afternoon to do the things you enjoy doing but don't often have time for.
- Window-shop with no agenda in a new city.
- Spend some time aimlessly in a used book store and find books that suit your interest.
- Create a new recipe, allow yourself to be creatively expressive.
- Browse through a museum with a notebook to note the things that pique your inner muse.
- Have a private picnic at a local park during your lunch hour.

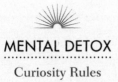

MENTAL DETOX
Curiosity Rules

To help you find ways to get into being more comfortable being alone and still with your thoughts, your mental detox is to spend time investigating and engaging your curiosity. Exploring the things that you find interesting will naturally carve out time to be quiet and still. Doing so will help throw a curveball to your daily rhythm of living in an electronically saturated and on-the-go society. As you explore these new interests, you will break the cycle of being mindlessly busy and will engage an area of your brain that is not often activated on a daily basis.

Make a list of three things that you have always been interested in learning more about but haven't had the time to investigate. Make a note in the space provided below, using the first line to write down your interest and the second line to identify why that particular thing is interesting to you. Over the next three days set aside twenty minutes each day to read or research these things about which you are curious. Imagine yourself as a child again, with an unquenchable curiosity, and allow yourself to keep asking yourself the question "why?" as you learn more and more about a subject that interests you. This active engagement of your curiosity will not only break previously existing mental patterns, but it will also fire up neurological triggers and rewards that will naturally encourage you to continue this exploratory learning process.

1) ....

2) ....

3) ....

4) ....

5) ....

6) ....

SPIRITUAL DETOX

Sharing Confidently

Since this new way gives us such confidence, we can
be very bold. (2 Corinthians 3:12)

Too many people feel alone in their faith because faith is not often openly talked about. Perhaps this is a result of people who are hypersensitive to being politically correct, or perhaps it is from a reluctance to discuss matters of the heart, but there is no reason not to talk openly about the most important thing in life: your heart and soul. What you believe in determines everything about your life; it is counterintuitive and contrary to living authentically not to talk about your faith. Faith is something that should bring us great joy, and that which brings us great joy should make us overflow with a desire to share that joy with others.

Share your joy by bringing up your relationship with Jesus Christ or with God at least three times today. Try to do so naturally and with confidence, even if you might feel hesitant or shy. As you speak more openly about your faith, you will find that people will be more receptive and open to you about theirs as well; as a result, you can live in a community of encouraging fellowship with others.

....

Father, show me areas in which I can slow my life down that I might be able to really connect with You and really engage in life. I want to learn how to value myself by who I am—and who You made me to be—instead of by how much I can accomplish or get done in a day. As I have more time to authentically connect with others, breathe into me boldness that I might be confident and open about where it is that my hope comes from. In the calming name of Jesus, Amen.

THE DESTINATION

The Truth: Life is about progress, not perfection.

Unfasten yourself from your Velcro attachment to the façade of perfection, and focus instead on celebrating your progress.

My Velcro Dog

I have a Velcro dog. No, that's not his breed; officially, Finnegan is an Irish terrier, a medium-sized ball of red wirehair and energy who is both fiercely independent and unable to be by himself. He's stubborn with an extra flare of determination. There are plenty of Velcro dog breeds, like golden retrievers and cocker spaniels, dogs who desperately want to be around their pack leaders to be snuggled and petted. Not Finnegan. Finnegan is Velcro in his need for affection but he's not affectionate—he has a jealous streak in him, an empty hole that gets larger anytime Brandon or I give love and attention to anything or anyone else.

Finnegan and Ellie are practically the same age; Finnegan was born the same week we found out that we were pregnant.

We welcomed Finn into our lives when he was just seven weeks old, and I was just seven weeks pregnant . . . tracking my pregnancy week-by-week alongside his puppy growth made for a wonderful and distraction-filled forty weeks. I was in nesting mode and so I treated Finnegan like my baby. He was practice for baby Ellie to come.

Irish terriers love babies and children. And Finnegan is no exception. He loves Ellie, but he is green-eyed over my blue-eyed baby. What he loves the most about her are her accessories. Impeccable in his timing, he stalks the house looking for blankets, hair bows, and her nasal bulb syringe anytime she starts crying. He knows crying leads to breastfeeding and breastfeeding leads to him being unsupervised. Freedom reigns. It is at that point he explores the house with mischievous intent.

And then starts the parade.

The metal tags on his dog collar jingle together as he stalks the hallways of the house searching for Ellie treasures. While I feed Ellie on the couch, Finn dashes around with his victories in tow. Obedient, he awaits the discipline of my firm "no" and immediately drops his most recent find. I am left with an array of blankets, stuffed animals, diapers, bows, hats, and sleepers sprawled across the living room and Finn is satisfied to have received the attention of discipline.

Finn is a work in progress. He is a little puppy in a big world and learning more and more every day how to become a better, more obedient dog. He is a dog though. He will never be perfect. No matter how mature he becomes or how well he outgrows his Velcro attachment for attention, he will still be a dog.

We're a lot like Finnegan: works in progress. And like the

limitations that come with being a dog, we have our own human limitations. We are human. We will never be perfect.

Life is a practice about progress, not perfection, a concept completely different from what the world tells us. We are told the lie that we can be perfect—that we can have the perfect body, the perfect family, the perfect job, and the perfect life. This pursuit of perfection puts us on an exhausting treadmill of achievement that has no end. One of the problems with the pursuit of perfect is that it removes us from our ability to be in the present moment and puts us in a state of hyperfocus on the future.

The best news of not having to pursue perfection is that it gives us permission to just live in the moment. The idea of perfection that consumes many of us is so far off in the future that it steals our ability to breathe and be alive in the now. Furthermore, living in the moment means that we can concentrate on what we do have control over: our training and our obedience. In the same way that Finnegan is trainable, we, too, are trainable.

Progress is achieved through training.

Unfasten yourself from your Velcro attachment to the façade of perfection. Train your brain and the flexibility of your mind every day by being committed to the "practice" and "training" of living. With the right training and intention, anyone can start seeing life from a positive perspective. The perspective with which you see the world—and your potential in it—is different based on whether your focus is on progress or on perfection.

In the same way that I celebrate Finnegan's victories of progress—the days when he heels well, when he sits on command, when he doesn't bark at the neighbor's dog, and when he plays by himself—we, too, must celebrate our victories. The more we celebrate the forward steps we take in life, the more forward steps we will actually take. Too often we hesitate to celebrate, wanting to wait for the finished product, but the reality is that there is no such thing as a finished product. Life is a progression of moments and opportunities; it is a journey, not a destination.

PHYSICAL DETOX
Celebrating Progress

We must get ourselves in the habit of celebration. I mean celebrations beyond weddings, special occasions, and birthdays. I firmly believe that we can find something to celebrate every day of our lives, weekdays as well as weekends. To help foster within you a heart of celebration, your physical detox is all about learning how to celebrate your body. Keeping in mind the lesson of this chapter—that progress itself is worthy of celebration—your physical detox is to celebrate yourself physically for the progress you have made over the past few years of your life.

Using the space provided below, write down three areas of progress that deserve to be acknowledged and celebrated. Things you can consider for celebration could include looking at yourself more kindly in the mirror, being more consistent in how often you take a walk with your friend or with your significant other, going to the gym more frequently, being able to move with more ease because you have been consistent with your morning stretches, feeling more refreshed or energized because you have implemented more sleep into your life, fitting better into your jeans thanks to a few weeks of cutting back on your sugar intake, or perhaps being resistant to whatever cold might be going around thanks to your strengthened immune system.

I celebrate the progress I have made physically in these areas:

....

....

....

....

....

....

MENTAL DETOX
Bold Proclamations

The phrase *It's the journey that matters, not the destination* is often quoted and well known, but not often well lived. It is much easier to recite this quotation than it is to live it out. As you consider how life is about progress, not perfection, you must also consider how you can actually live out that truth instead of just knowing about it. Knowledge is not true knowledge until it is put into application. This mental detox of setting bold proclamations is intended to start helping you put this knowledge into true application.

In the spaces provided below, write out five bold proclamations, starting with the phrase *I love the journey of my life because . . .* to help you really celebrate the beautiful things that make the journey more important than the destination.

I love the journey of my life because

....

I love the journey of my life because

....

I love the journey of my life because

....

I love the journey of my life because

....

I love the journey of my life because

....

SPIRITUAL DETOX

Obedient Follow Through

You must love the Lord your God and always obey his requirements, decrees, regulations, and commands. (Deuteronomy 11:1)

Finnegan's obedience is sometimes reluctant, but it is still obedience when he follows through and listens to my commands. I have structure set in place for Finnegan for his own good and with his best interest at heart. I celebrate when Finn obeys. And God celebrates when we obey Him, too.

What is one area of your life in which you have not been fully obedient to God? Perhaps you have always known you should love others more radically and with more generosity as God commanded, but you haven't yet taken action on doing so. Perhaps you have always thought about tithing or giving more money away to others, but haven't yet followed through. Perhaps you know that you are commanded to forgive others as you have been forgiven, yet you are still holding on to a grudge or have a heart filled with resentment and anger. Or perhaps you are aware of a sinful habit in which you engage that you don't want to stop. Whatever it might be for you, there are many ways each of us can be more obedient to the principles of God and the teachings of Jesus.

Identify where in your heart you can be more obedient to God and follow through on that obedience, with a cheerful heart, starting today.

....

*Father, I know that life is about the journey and
not the destination, but I so often get distracted
by the focus on the destination that I lose myself
in the journey. Teach me how to live differently.
Remind me to pursue excellence, not perfection,
every day and empower me with wisdom to be
able to live consciously in the present moment.
In the everlasting name of Jesus, Amen.*

INCOMPLETENESS

The Truth: God is the ultimate Validator in your life.

We were created with a God-sized hole in our hearts that nothing but He can fill.

God-Sized Hole

Rainy days at the beach were reserved for a few things: reading on the porch, eating ice cream for lunch, and spending the afternoon putting a jigsaw puzzle together. My grandma and I always teamed up as partners. It was our job to find the edges and corners. We did serious jigsaw puzzles. Thousand-piece ones. Ones with complicated photographs, and sometimes those that had edges with multiple possibilities.

The kitchen table hosted our chaotic spread of pieces and we passed hours finding a home for each one. Despite our most careful effort to keep each puzzle's pieces intact in its box, occasionally we found ourselves in a puzzlers' nightmare: a completed puzzle with just one piece missing. After hours of tedious effort the open puzzle hole mocked us. There was nothing that could be done. No way to fill that hole. No way to complete that puzzle.

An incomplete puzzle, no matter how close to completion, is never complete. In the same way, an incomplete heart, no matter how close to completion, is never complete. I should know, I lived for years with an incomplete heart.

An incomplete heart is one that is close to happiness, but can't quite arrive. It is one that knows there is great purpose to life, yet can't quite find its place. It is a heart that flickers with the hope of meaning, when it knows that the full blaze of a flame is possible. These incomplete hearts aren't our fault— we were created with them; we were created with a hole in us. It is a God-sized hole. It is a hole that cannot be filled with anything other than Him, though it is in our human nature to try. The hole will always be there—God Himself put it there—and it is there to remind us on a daily basis that we need Him. Everyone has this God-sized hole. There are dozens of ways we try to fill that hole—perfectionism, food, drugs, sex, control, wealth, acceptance, achievement—that will never fill the void. Only God can fill the God-sized hole.

I have tried to fill this hole on my own. The hole made me ache and so I sought to dull it. I started numbing the emptiness with achievement, winning athletic accolades and racking up an armory of trophies to prove my worth and value. I still felt the ache. Next I indulged my affinity for control and developed my perfectionism, assuming that I could perfect my life on my own and that as I did, the hole would close up. When the hole didn't disappear, I poured more of myself into it. I filled myself up by emptying my stomach and pursuing an ideal body, telling myself that the ache would go away when I just finally lost those last five pounds. The five pounds came and went and my heart felt the same. The happiness I expected to come never came. I masked my emotion and my pain by filling the hole with the distraction of my eating disorder. I changed my outlook and focused on climbing the corporate ladder, making more money and becoming more popular, as those things would surely fill some of the emptiness of the ache. The money, success, and alcohol that came as a result only made me feel emptier and achier. No matter how hard I tried and no matter what I tried, I could not fill the hole. I knew I was so close to being complete and so close to being happy, like a jigsaw puzzle being just one piece short of completion, but I couldn't seem to find or create the missing puzzle piece.

Finally, after I exhausted my resources, and myself, I gave my soul the puzzle piece it craved: God.

I had known God before, and known Him well, but I hadn't walked with Him in a way that would fill the hole. As a kid I always knew that God loved me, and I loved Him, but I didn't really connect with Him as being foundational to my happiness and joy. He was a bonus, an important one, but not the full source of where I found my validation.

The God-sized hole in my heart is the piece of me from where my validation and worth comes. When filled, I know I am complete. I know I am good enough. I know I am lovely. I know I have purpose. I know I have worth. I know I have a life worth telling a story about. I know I am loved. I know I am enough.

We were designed to crave God, yet many of us do not know how to really connect with Him—to deeply connect— in order to fill that craving. As an adult, once I had exhausted all of my desperate attempts to fill the hole on my own, I had to relearn how to have a relationship with God. I learned that I needed Him daily. I learned that I needed to spend the first five minutes of my day with Him in quiet prayer, reflection, and reading. I learned that my days are better when I start them with worship music and singing. I learned that my mind comes alive when I listen to sermons or uplifting spiritual podcasts while I fold laundry and empty the dishwasher. I learned that God walks with me in the smallness of my days and because of that I learned just how much He cares about the small things. I learned how much He cares for me and I learned to trust Him more. I learned to surrender control. I learned to believe that He is for me, not against me. I learned to talk about Him more. I learned to live with confidence in who He made me to be and with contentment about where He put me to be. In short, I learned that God is real, that He is alive and that He really does care about me.

This new understanding of His love gave me permission to stop trying so hard to impress others. It gave me freedom to be my best in life, not to prove myself or earn value, but rather to make the most of what I have been given. It is God's love that fills my hole. It is His love that gives me greater joy and happiness than I could have ever imagined possible. It is His love that pieces all of the pain of my life together to make a beautiful work of art. It is His love that takes my rainy days of life and makes them lovely.

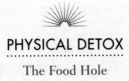

PHYSICAL DETOX
The Food Hole

As I mentioned, I tried to fill my God-sized hole with food. Food became my source of comfort in a variety of ways, sometimes in ways that were controlled and sometimes that were out of control. During the years I struggled with a binge-eating disorder, I turned to food when anxious, filling my stomach as much as I could to numb and distract myself from the emotional pain I was experiencing. At the opposite end of the spectrum, to make up for these overindulgences, I spent days after a binge cycling through food restriction and purging habits. My relationship with food was like a swinging pendulum, always moving from one extreme to the other, passing through the middle point of balance, but not often resting there.

There are millions of people who have turned to food for comfort in ways similar to my experience. While many of these people may not have a clinically diagnosable eating disorder, they do suffer from disordered eating habits, or a negative and unhealthy relationship with food. A negative relationship with food can make you feel out of control, cause unwanted weight gain (or prevent wanted weight loss), and intensify emotional anxiety. A positive relationship with food allows the person to eat well, indulge in moderation, and maintain a healthy and ideal body weight.

Assess your relationship with food by taking just a minute to reflect on the role of food in your life. You may have a negative relationship with food if you answer "yes" to any of the following questions:

> Do you obsess about your calorie intake?
>
> Do you ever skip meals on purpose?
>
> Do you ever feel guilt associated with food that you have eaten?
>
> Do you ascribe food to certain categories, being "good" or "bad"?
>
> Do you ever eat to the point of your stomach hurting?
>
> Do you struggle to stop eating once you have had enough?
>
> Do you turn to food when emotionally stressed or upset?
>
> Do you engage in nighttime eating?
>
> Do you have short periods of overeating, or bingeing?
>
> Do you think about food all day long?
>
> Do you eliminate entire food categories such as carbohydrates?
>
> Do you have fear about letting go of a controlled diet?

The good news is that as in all relationships, the relationship you have with food is one that you *can* develop in a positive way each and every day. Invest in your relationship with food today for your physical detox by honestly assessing the health of your relationship. Next, identify in which area the relationship feels most out of balance and create a short journal entry on your phone for the next seven days to simply track how that specific area is going. By simply being aware of where your relationship with food is toxic or negative you can start improving the relationship and empowering yourself to change the relationship for the better.

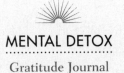

MENTAL DETOX
Gratitude Journal

Gratitude journaling is a transformational personal habit that not only sets your mind up with an attitude of gratitude for the rest of the day, but also lines the God-sized hole in your heart with thankfulness.

You can customize your style of gratitude journaling to suit whatever your preferences are, but people who have the most success with a gratitude journal are those who have created their own specific and special journal. This journal can be an electronic app on your phone or it can be a physical journal dedicated to handwriting out your gratitude list. When you journal, make a list of ten to twelve things for which you are grateful for at that moment. These things should be the first things that pop into your mind, and whether they are big or small, they're worth noting.

Start your habit of gratitude journaling today. Plan to do it as part of your morning routine before you leave the house, or keep it on your desk at the office and do it before you check your email each day. By making your gratitude journal a cornerstone of your mornings, you will pave the way for a good rest of the day.

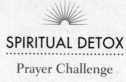

SPIRITUAL DETOX

Prayer Challenge

Devote yourselves to prayer with an alert mind and a thankful heart. (Colossians 4:2)

A hole in many people's spiritual walk is found in their prayer life. We often use prayer as a last resort instead of as our first action because we have failed to create a consistent prayer life with God.

Your prayer challenge is to add the habit of saying a small prayer of gratitude every day after you complete your gratitude journal. This will get you in the habit of praying not just for things or when you are in need. It will help you connect to God daily in conversation at the start of your day and then it will be easier to reconnect with Him throughout the rest of your day.

....

Father, I praise You for the God-sized hole You put inside of me, for it reminds me daily of my need for You. Forgive me for the ways in which I have tried to fill that hole, and my needs, without You. Thank You for being my ultimate Validator and for making me complete. In the name of Jesus, the One who enables my full completion and connection with You, Amen.

EXTERNAL AFFIRMATION

The Truth: Real life happens when
you walk your own path.

The more we chase a destination of achievement, the more that
destination changes, creating a moving finish line . . . a race of
life that is exhausting and keeps us from really living.

Moving Finish Lines

As a competitive runner, I am familiar with racing varying distances, ranging from a 5K to a full marathon. I prefer marathons; however, for effective training, it is important for me to race the shorter distances as well. A few years back, my coach signed me up for an 8K race, a distance I didn't know anything about until I got to the start line at seven a.m. on a foggy summer morning.

I'm the girl at the start line who likes to talk to everyone. It keeps my nerves down and prevents me from thinking too much about the race itself. In typical fashion, I gathered information from fellow runners about the course and made a strategic plan in my head against my competition. This race had prize money at stake and I love winning prizes. Not knowing the converted distance of an 8K into miles, and not having a calculator on hand, I asked around and ascertained that it was *about* four miles long.

Eager to win, I pushed myself hard. I decided to try to maintain my short-distance threshold speed, a pace I usually reserved for the 3.1-mile distance of a 5K. If I could run a specific pace for 3.1 miles, why couldn't I maintain it for a mere 0.9 miles more? It was going to be painful and tough, but it was certain to give me victory and prize money, making it worth the discomfort.

I approached what I thought was the final half-mile of the race exhausted, but thinking the finish line was around the corner gave me an emotional burst that I translated into even more speed. At my fastest pace possible, I held on for dear life as I pushed my body and anticipated the finish line. The course wove in and out of downtown street blocks, and with every turn I expected it to arrive. It didn't. There was no finish line in sight.

The four-mile mark passed. Lactic acid started to weigh down my legs and extreme fatigue set in. I was positive the course had been improperly measured. The turns kept coming. Cramping set into my legs. When the four-and-a-half-mile mark arrived, I shouted angrily at onlookers, asking them where the finish line was. I was told that I was "almost there" and it was *just* another half-mile away.

With heavy legs and an even heavier heart I finally crossed the finish line at 4.97 miles, which, as it turns out is the exact distance of an 8K. I had been misinformed. I had created a race with a moving finish line.

Anything in life can be turned into a moving finish line

when chased with the wrong attitude. When we strive to achieve for the sake of affirmation or to build our perceived worth, we set ourselves up for an exhausting race in life. We exhaust ourselves running races with moving finish lines as we try to earn approval, status, success, and acceptance. The pursuit takes us on a journey with a moving finish line. The closer we get to what we think we want, the further away the mark moves. Even though we know that impressing others will never earn us the approval and meaning that our souls so desperately crave, we still chase the moving finish lines of their opinions and standards.

In addition to the cases of moving finish lines in *racing,* there are also instances in *our lives* in which we similarly feel like we've crossed the "finish line" and then it, too, disappears. In such cases, we have set a goal and achieved it. We have climbed the mountain and enjoyed the triumph. We have overcome a bad habit and created a good one in its place. These finishes permit us to experience great elation, joy, and accomplishment. They put us on top of the world. But eventually the high wears off. Our joy fades. We tire of the view from that particular mountaintop. This is known as the What Now? syndrome. It is a different type of moving finish line. It's a finish line that we have told ourselves will fulfill us, yet after we cross it, we find ourselves still lacking and still wanting more.

I've experienced the What Now? syndrome in a variety of ways. During my years of disordered eating, when I finally reached my unhealthy goal weight, it didn't feel as good as I thought it would. My What Now? became the pursuit of an even lower number on the scale. When I climbed the corporate ladder, I only yearned to be promoted again and to climb even higher. When I completed my first world championship triathlon event, I wanted to qualify for even more and to perform even better. When I experienced a major financial breakthrough and increased my earnings, I wanted to make even more money. The more money I made, the more money I felt I needed to make. The more athletic achievements I accomplished, the more athletic achievements I felt I needed. The more success I experienced, the more success I needed.

The What Now? syndrome is common to us all. It's the feeling we get when we finally get what we want and we then ask ourselves: *Is there more to life than this? Is this all there is?*

There is more to life. I have learned this lesson the hard way. The meaning and satisfaction I have searched for so desperately from life didn't come from where I thought it would. The achievements didn't fulfill me; they actually left me feeling empty and unfulfilled, wanting more. My soul became satisfied when I turned my heart to something more long-lasting: the legacy my life would leave. And I learned that the only way to leave a legacy that mattered was to really make a difference in the lives of others. I didn't need to impress others anymore, instead I needed to love them and be someone who improved the quality of their lives.

The thing about finish lines is that the line will always keep moving as long as we find our affirmation in external things. They will keep moving until we stop looking for impressiveness in what we do and instead find our impressiveness in who we are.

You can slow down your exhausting pace. You don't have to try so hard. You don't have to live in discomfort, always wondering about being good enough. The race of your life isn't being timed. There is a prize though, but it's not like a typical race. The prize isn't given to the person who finishes the fastest; it is given to all who run their race well. It is within the moments of the race itself that the prize exists—the ability to savor life as it is happening and appreciate each experience with great pleasure and joy. The ultimate achievement of life isn't in what or how much we achieve, it is in living fully within the pursuit of our achievements.

It's time to stop chasing and start living. Remove yourself from the never-ending rat race of approval and just run your own race. Your race doesn't have a finish line—it only has a path: to enjoy God as He enjoys you, and to love others.

PHYSICAL DETOX
Plank Power

As we journey along the pathway of our lives, our bodies need physical strength and endurance. Strengthen your core endurance by doing the plank hold. The plank hold is widely considered the most effective core exercise for the body, promoting toned stomach muscles, the reduction of low-back pain, and improvement of overall balance and posture.

To perform a plank hold, put yourself in a push-up position, with the front of your body prone, or facing the floor. Position yourself on your toes and hold your body up by resting on your palms with straightened elbows or on your forearms with bent elbows. Keep the height of your shoulders in line with the height of your hips, making a table out of your body. Engage your stomach, or core muscles by tightening your gluteal muscles and by pulling your belly button toward your spine. Once in position, simply hold the pose as long as you can.

Try to start with holding the plank position for a period of 20 seconds, and then increase weekly by adding an additional 5 seconds to challenge yourself. Build your endurance up to two sets of 60- to 90-second plank holds per day. Take a break from reading and try a plank hold right now. Time yourself and see how long you can hold the plank while maintaining good form.

MENTAL DETOX
Comparison Cut

One of the influences that kept me racing, in vain, toward a constantly moving finish line was the act of comparing myself to others. This is a common theme for many people, as we live in a culture of constant comparison. As a result, the finish lines of our lives often move because we are constantly looking around at the races of others.

Your mental detox is to cut the comparisons out of your life. Stop constantly comparing yourself to others by being like a racehorse—run your race with blinders on. Your metaphorical blinders are going to be intentional reminders to block out what other people are doing and to instead use your energy and focus to look forward at your own path.

For the purpose of this detox, your blinders will be a rubber band or hair tie. Cut comparison out of your mind by wearing the rubber band or hair tie on your wrist for the next three days and pull it any time you mentally catch yourself engaging in a comparison to someone else. This exercise isn't intended to eliminate mental comparisons completely, simply to help you start becoming more aware of the frequency in which you engage in them. Once you know how to catch the comparative thoughts, you will then be able to start replacing them with thoughts that are focused on what matters—that is, on thoughts about running your own race.

SPIRITUAL DETOX
Enjoying God

We know how much God loves us, and we have put our trust in his love. God is love, and all who live in love live in God, and God lives in them. (1 John 4:16)

If what we are looking for in life isn't found in the achievement of measurable successes, but rather, in the accomplishment of living beautifully, then we must find a way to really live well. I have found that the best way to live well is to find my pleasure in God and in His presence in my life. It has taken me time to learn how to enjoy God, but as soon as I learned that He always has my best intentions at heart, I found that I was then free to enjoy all that He has given me and put into my life.

To really enjoy God, you first must trust Him; trust that He is *for* you, and *not against* you. As you establish trust in His goodness, you will find yourself surrounded with an increased awareness of all of the good He has put into your life. Then, the more you enjoy God, the more you will trust Him. The more you trust Him, the more you will feel free to be yourself. The more you are yourself, the more you will be capable of pouring into the lives of others. The more you trust your worth, the less time you will spend trying to prove yourself to others, and the more capacity you will have to be alive and fully engaged in your journey of life.

Take a moment today to thank God for five things you really enjoy about your life right now. Thank Him for allowing those things, people, or experiences to be in your life and thank Him for giving you the capacity to enjoy them, and ultimately to enjoy Him. Fill in your five things in the space provided below:

....

....

....

....

....

....

Father, it is so easy for me to get distracted by others in life and I so easily compare my journey to theirs. Break me from this destructive habit and from my desire for external affirmation. Let the only affirmation I care about be that of Yours. Give me the boldness I need to walk the path You have set before me. In the beautiful name of Jesus, Amen.

DISTORTED PERCEPTION

The Truth: You can choose the right perspective in life.

Our perceptions in life do not always align with the realities of what is really going on, but with the right intentional thinking you can shift your perspective at any moment.

Dolphin Attack

Surfing is one of the most peaceful activities I enjoy. I like to consider myself a surfer even though I don't live by the ocean, didn't grow up in a surf culture, and only picked up the sport at age twenty-nine. Surfing called to me: it was as if the ocean waves sang a lullaby luring me into them. It didn't make sense to get involved in a sport that you can't do on a consistent basis, but when your heart speaks, you must listen. When I do get to surf, the world disappears: it's just my surfboard, the ocean, me, and God. Oh, and sharks.

After I bought my first board, a brand-new pink-marbled Hawaiian classic, I couldn't wait to go surfing. The closest beach was a three-hour drive away. My heart dictated the melody of my mood, though, and all I could think about once I got my own board was getting on it. My mind was consumed. I just absolutely had to get myself to the ocean.

In an effort to be in the water at the peak of sunrise, I found myself happily on the road at 3:15 a.m. The feeling of being in the water as pink rays of light stretched across the surface was like receiving a present from God. The waves were wonderful and bigger than usual for Virginia Beach. The surf report had predicted a flat ocean so I found myself alone in the waters that God had prepared for me. The waves crashed for me alone upon the empty beach. It was beautifully peaceful and so worth my early-morning drive.

Then a lull occurred. The waves subsided. And then it happened.

A gray fin broke the surface no more than fifteen yards from me. I was isolated. I was far from shore. No one was on the beach and no one knew I was out surfing.

Panic filled my heart. I shook on my board as my body throbbed, bringing more attention to myself in the empty ocean. The fin surfaced again. Closer this time. I bit my lip to hold back my tears.

An eternity of minutes passed as I floated frozen in fear. The ocean rocked me back and forth as my mind prepared for the worst.

The fin reappeared, but it undulated this time. Rhythmically it continued, and then a few more fins joined in its dance. In a moment of realization, a tear of joy escaped my eye—I was surrounded by a school of dolphins, *not* sharks.

My initial perception—that of being in shark-infested waters—was not the reality of what happened that morning, even though emotionally I experienced it as if it had been. What I experienced was a suspended reality in which my perception was my reality. It was a classic example of the psychological phenomenon that whatever we perceive to be real is what we experience as real. The way we assess the world is the way we will experience the world.

Our perceptions in life do not always align with the realities of what is really going on. We have limited vision that is often blurred or distorted. Much of what deepens the roots of our insecurities are misperceived and misaligned perspectives about who we really are and what we are really experiencing. We can detox this insecurity by simply reframing the perspective with which we see the world.

You can learn to hone your perspective skills. The key to being able to adjust your perspective is the initial knowledge that you are actually in control of it. With the right intentional thinking you can shift your perspective at any moment and during any situation.

Here are some practical ways in which you can practice painting your mind with the perspective of your choice:

- *Be active minded.* Choose to have an *actively* engaged perspective—not a passive one. Your mind is accustomed to thinking a certain way, and often this is in a negative way, so naturally your perspective will be slanted in that direction. An active mind makes deliberate choices in what it chooses to see and focus on.
- *Know the power of your thoughts.* What you believe to be true will be true. So, if your thoughts are overwhelmingly negative, you will lead a negative life and suffer emotionally. If your

thoughts are focused on the positive, opportunities and happiness will unfold before you.

- *Search for truth.* Ask yourself, "Is this thought true?" and "Is there a way to know that it is absolutely true?" By becoming a truth-seeker, you will become more sensitive to identifying untruths and being able to combat them from lingering in your mind.
- *Be proactive.* Approach a daunting obstacle with vigor instead of with dread—resist the temptation to put it off and do it right away.
- *Create a "get to" mind-set.* One simple mental filter that can successfully fine-tune the vocabulary of your mind is to filter out your use of the phrase "have to." Instead of "having to" do something substitute the "have" with the word "get" and you will begin "getting to" the positive opportunities that abound in your life. This simple shift of word choice can shift your entire perspective and your experience of your day-to-day tasks.
- *Focus on the present.* Most people are in a perpetual state of partial attention—and because of this split attention, most people lose their present moments to obsessing over their past or their future. Spend your mental energy thinking about the present moment that is right in front of you, *not* on what happened in the past or what might happen in the future.
- *Expect that all will be well.* Life will be full of curveballs—unexpected circumstances, finan-

cial worry, emotional pain, physical sickness, disappointment, and general hurt—but the triumphant mind knows that no matter what happens, all will be well. Those with this type of perspective have high expectations of life and of others—not necessarily that everything will happen as expected or anticipated—but rather, that no matter how things play out, in all things, God causes everything to work together for the good of those who love Him. (Romans 8:28)

- *Be big-minded.* Being big-minded is the same as being big-souled—that is, having an attitude that God is great and that His story of glory will prevail through your life no matter what happens. Life will have problems, but a big-minded person knows that God is always bigger than any problem or hurt or pain that can exist.

Perspective changes everything. We can ultimately step away from our insecurities when we are willing to adjust our perspective about the world around us. Refuse to see yourself surrounded by sharks in life when more often than not you are in the midst of a playful school of dolphins.

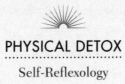

PHYSICAL DETOX

Self-Reflexology

Feet, an often-overlooked part of the body, are the foundation of all movement. They support our weight, they take us places, and they connect us to the ground. Taking care of your feet is an important element of taking care of your overall physical health. Your physical detox for this chapter is to spend some time and attention on the care of your feet, specifically through reflexology. Reflexology, the application of specific pressure to hands and feet, is an ancient art and alternative therapy method originating in Chinese and Egyptian cultures.

In your personal self-reflexology therapy you are going to use a simple tennis ball, lacrosse ball, or golf ball. From a standing position, place your ball of choice under one of your feet and gently apply body-weight pressure onto that foot, pressing your foot into the ball. Glide and roll the ball back and forth along your foot, from the top of the toes to the bottom of the heel. Be sure to tilt your foot inwardly as well in order to allow the ball to hit pressure points along the inner arch of your foot. Finish your reflexology session by spending a minute making small circles with the ball around the surface area of the heel. Once you have performed this upon one foot—which should take about two minutes in total—switch feet and repeat the process.

As you work on each foot, know that the work you do on your left foot will correspond to a benefit for the left side of your body and all of your organs and valves found there, and vice versa for the right side of your body. Incorporate self-reflexology at least three times per week for healthy feet and a healthy body.

MENTAL DETOX
Anxious Antidotes

Anxiety doesn't have to have a place of permanence in our perspective. The experience of anxiety can make you feel like your head is surrounded by fog, distracting your thoughts with clouds of uneasiness. Anxiety distorts our perception of reality; it allows us to believe that we are surrounded by sharks when in fact we are actually in the midst of dolphins.

In particular, social anxiety is a not often talked about struggle that plagues many people. The good news is that social anxiety can be pacified with the right tools. To overcome social anxiety, employ this strategic approach: identify the last person you were nervous to talk to or be around. When you think about that interaction try to remember exactly what it was about them or that scenario that brought you anxiety, or that caused you to feel insecure or engulfed with self-doubt. As you think about the specifics, identify *why* you wanted that person, or group of people, to like you. Also, *what* was it that you hoped to get out of that conversation or interaction?

Understanding *why* you are anxious will help you better shift your understanding and perspective on *being* anxious. When I finally realized that I felt anxious around people I admired, I was better able to control my anxiety because I realized the anxiety wasn't about me at all. Instead, it was a yearning for validation from people whom I esteemed. Instead of dwelling on something I could not control—someone else's opinion of me—I now channel my anxious energy to focusing on exactly what it is about that person that I so admire and want to emulate. Identifying what I admire about others allows me to have a positive perspective as I interact with them.

With the right shift in perspective you can channel anxiety into a productive emotion that promotes your personal development and growth. By stopping and assessing the cause and root of the anxiety you experience, rather than dwelling on the experience of anxiety itself, you can find freedom. The next time you feel social anxiety start to itch inside of you, causing you to feel uncertain of yourself or a situation, channel your perspective into something that will produce a positive outcome. Remind yourself that everyone feels insecure and uncertain at times and that such feelings do not always reflect the truth. It's okay to feel anxious; it's not okay to let that anxiety win.

SPIRITUAL DETOX

Recalling Rescues

"Lord, help!" they cried in their trouble, and he saved them from their distress. (Psalm 107:28)

There is nothing like thinking you are going to die to make you appreciate being alive. In my case, even though I was among dolphins and not sharks, I still felt rescued by God when I safely exited the waters that day. The relief that we experience in these moments of rescue is a taste of what grace is.

Recall a difficult time in your life. After you do so, freeze the framework of that memory and re-imagine yourself in those circumstances. Since hindsight is 20/20, consider the situation from a macro perspective and compare that to the micro perspective that you most likely had while you were living the scenario. Next, since you know how the story ends and how you were ultimately rescued or healed from the difficulty, try to visualize God's presence in the darkness that you possibly couldn't see prior.

....

Father, I submit to You my perspective, that You might help me always see life from the right perspective and with the right attitude, knowing that You are good and that You are always working things together for my good. I may not understand the circumstances and challenges of my life, but I do understand and believe that You are good. Thank You for taking everything in my life and using it for good. In the good name of Jesus, Amen.

THE MIRROR

The Truth: God sees you as perfect.

*We can learn to see ourselves as He sees us by first
knowing that the mirror we see is broken.*

Fuzzy-Eye Syndrome

My house is filled with elephants, stuffed ones. Ellie loves elephants, so I seem to add more to the collection with every
week that passes. To be fair, Ellie didn't have a choice in the
matter—we themed her nursery around elephants with hues
of light pink and gray accents, and I made a concerted effort
to purchase every dress, blanket, bib, and pacifier in existence
that had elephants on it.

It all started when we decided on her name: Ellie. In my
heart I just knew that a little girl named Ellie would love elephants, or her little "Ellies" as we call them in our house.
Ellie and I have even ridden an elephant—an elephant
named Beautiful—when she was just twenty-two weeks in
the womb. Ellie is too young to take to the circus just yet to

see a real live elephant, but that day will come soon and I can't wait.

I'm comfortable with circuses, too comfortable perhaps—I spent years of my life feeling like I was living at a circus. My life was filled with circus funhouse mirrors. The way I saw myself—in my mirrored reflection and in my mind—was as lopsided and loopy as the distorting effects of the convex and concave mirrors of the circus. Even though I was fit, healthy, and at an ideal weight for my body, the image I saw in the mirror was the opposite. I saw myself the size of an elephant. My eyes exaggerated my "problem areas." My mind construed the reflection with a negative filter, always looking for something about which to be upset. I felt huge and uncomfortable in my skin. My eyes didn't see me for who I really was or for how I really looked. When I looked at myself I didn't recognize myself. My reflection became a stranger to me and I became a stranger to myself. Eventually, I started avoiding mirrors, anxious about the image that I might see. My body dysmorphia was not something I shared with anyone—it made me feel crazy, like I really did belong on display at a circus or as part of the freak show, but as I later learned, I was not alone. Millions of people struggle with a negative body image in the same way that I did, it's just that no one talks about it.

There's something I learned recently about elephants that makes me love them even more than I did when I first decided that Ellie would love elephants. Elephants are one of the few animals that can recognize their own reflection in mirrors. Mirrors don't lie to elephants the way they lied to me.

Many of us have lived too long in a circus-mirror world. We have settled for a distorted view of ourselves, and unlike elephants, we spend years of our lives not knowing what we actually look like. We don't see ourselves physically for just how beautiful we are and for how amazing and miraculous our bodies are. Even worse, we don't see ourselves clearly on the inside for the potential, purpose, and worth we really have.

The day the mirror straightened out for me was the day I finally realized that I needed to zoom out the lens of my eyes. I needed to start looking at myself as a whole instead of as a half or as parts that I didn't like. Previously, I had a bad habit of only focusing on what I didn't like in the mirror. My critical eye was immediately drawn to whatever body part I was unhappy with. I pulled and picked myself apart and found myself spending an inordinate amount of time focusing on what I liked least about my body and my personality, ultimately making those negative things the only things I could see in my own reflection. What we focus on always becomes larger in our lives, and for me that meant that the little things I didn't like about myself became colossal, taking up a large portion of my mental and emotional thought-space.

The truth is that without God's mirror we all have a distorted view of ourselves. What we see in the mirror is not what God sees. Our mirror is broken. The cracks come from the sin, the hurt, and the pain of life, and together they shatter our ability to see clearly. It's hard on our own to see ourselves for who we really are—for who God created us to be. God sees the real us. He sees us as His precious children. We are perfect in His eyes and He is able to see in us what we cannot see. We can learn to see ourselves as He sees us by first knowing that the mirror we see is broken.

We see flaws. God sees perfection.

We see insecurity. God sees confidence.

We see fear. God sees faith.

We see limitations. God sees limitlessness.

We see our scars. God sees healing.

We see mistakes. God sees lessons.

We see blemishes. God sees beauty.

We see uncertainty. God sees certainty.

We see averageness. God sees uniqueness.

We see doubt. God sees worth.

We see dullness. God sees potential and purpose.

We see awkwardness. God sees where we fit.

When we understand that the mirror we are looking into is broken, we can arrive more quickly at a place of kindness toward ourselves. We have the option of looking into a different mirror—into God's mirror. The day I realized that it was my mirror that was broken, not me, was the day that my self-worth transformed. It was that day that I decided to switch mirrors. In my mirror I am broken, but in God's mirror I am whole. In His mirror I am perfect. In His mirror I am beautiful. In His mirror I have great purpose, worth, and potential. In His mirror I am enough. In His mirror I matter. Our reflection in God's mirror is the only reflection that matters.

Trust God's mirror. Even if you can't see it, His mirror is the only mirror that matters. And as you learn to see yourself as He sees you, you will become more like an elephant in the good sense . . . in the sense that you can finally see yourself for the uniquely amazing and beautiful creation that you are, recognizing yourself as God recognizes you.

PHYSICAL DETOX
....
Fuzzy Fitness Expectations

Most people who have failed to reach their fitness goals haven't fallen short because of a lack of effort, but rather because they had fuzzy, undefined expectations. If you don't set goals for yourself, you don't have a goal to work toward. Likewise, if you aren't sure what your ideal level of health and wellness looks like, you won't be motivated to pursue, achieve, or maintain it on a daily basis.

Decide what health looks like to you.

> How active would you like to be?
> What is your body's happy and healthy set point
>   weight?
> What sort of physical activities would you like to be
>   able to do with your family?
> When you consider yourself and your future into
>   your old age, what would you like to be able to
>   do physically with your grandchildren?
> How do you expect your body to age?

Use the space provided below to answer the preceding questions so that you don't have fuzzy expectations about your health and fitness. The clearer you set your expectations, the better results you will get and the more control you will have over your health.

- I want to be physically active .... days per week.

- My body's natural and happy body weight is ....
- I most enjoy doing .... and ....
  as physical exercise.
- I am committed to eating more ....
  and more .... in my diet so that my
  body continues to age well.
- When I have grandchildren I would like to be
  able to do .... and
  .... with them and show them
  how to live an active life by my example.

MENTAL DETOX
Social Media Sabbatical

One of the reasons we don't see ourselves for who we really are is because we are overly concerned about others, about what they are doing and about what they think about us. The fuzzy eyes with which we see ourselves are often a by-product of the social media culture in which we live. While social media has a lot of positive benefits in connecting us to others, it also has the potential to be detrimental to our mental and emotional health. It becomes toxic when it takes our focus off of our own lives and puts it on the lives of others.

Give your mind a mental break and take a sabbatical from social media for at least three full days. Eliminate one major form of social media from your life, starting today as soon as you finish reading this paragraph. If you have the corresponding app on your phone, delete the app completely—don't trust yourself to have willpower to not scroll through newsfeeds when you are bored or passing time. To take this mental detox to the next level, disconnect from all forms of social media for all three days. As you take your social media sabbatical, use the time you would normally spend on social media and invest it in doing something you really enjoy, like taking a walk, trying out a new recipe, or reading a book. This sabbatical will help you clear your mind from the clutter of comparison and will give you a clearer ability to see yourself and your life without a fuzzy filter.

SPIRITUAL DETOX

Voicing Praise

It is good to give thanks to the Lord, to sing praises to the Most High. (Psalm 92:1)

We have the ability to change the way we see our reflection by changing the way we think. As you have learned, changing our thoughts takes time, but one way to start making deposits into developing that positive change is by speaking praises, or words of affirmation, with more frequent intention. By voicing praise and being someone of kind words, we can build up the confidence of not only those around us, but of ourselves as well. The more we train our minds to speak words of life, the more naturally words of life will come to the forefront of our thoughts.

Be a positive mirror for others by seizing the opportunity to speak praise anytime you think something kind or complimentary about someone. Too often we have a habit of thinking kind things, but not voicing them out loud. Speak them immediately. Words of affirmation can be life changing and eye opening; we all need them.

Be uplifting in your words toward others and in doing so you will be someone who helps others see themselves as God sees them. Your kind words and compliments can help clear up the fuzzy vision that others have of themselves. The more you love in this way, the more you will feel love yourself. Additionally, the more you help others see themselves as God sees them, the more you will be able to see yourself as God sees you. Make it your intention today to shower at least five people in your life with purposeful compliments and affirmations.

....

Father, thank You for creating me to look the way I do. You see beauty in me that I sometimes can't see and I praise You for loving me so completely. Teach me how to borrow Your eyes and how to start seeing myself as You see me, that I might not be dragged down or distracted by insecurities I feel about my physical appearance. In the perfect name of Jesus, Amen.

PERFECTIONISTIC THINKING

*The Truth: You don't have to strive for perfection;
you just have to strive to be yourself.*

Perfectionism separates us from contentment, but you can break the cycle of perfectionism by flooding yourself with the truth of what God says about you.

Puncturing Perfectionism

They say opposites attract. I didn't believe it until the day my handsome husband carried me across the threshold of our house after our honeymoon. That's when my perfect bubble popped.

It all started when we unpacked the moving truck. I discovered that Brandon had boxes upon boxes of man-cave treasures that simply didn't meet my standards. Broken trophies, souvenir shot glasses, beer signage, tacky posters, moldy T-shirts, and otherwise nondescript college memorabilia. As the U-Haul truck emptied further, smelly and stained furniture appeared that I had never seen. He had kept it all from his fraternity days in college, a good fifteen years prior. Thankfully, most everything ended up in the garage. After a few months there, they made their way to Goodwill.

But the boxes and furniture were just my first clue.

As we settled into our newlywed pace of life together, I noticed a fundamental crack between what we each considered down time. Brandon was able to sit for hours. He took his time doing his honey-do list, never stressing about what did or didn't get done. He approached tasks thoroughly, but not compulsively or obsessively.

My down time is different. It always involves an ambitious to-do list, a cup of dark coffee or espresso, and high-energy music to keep my momentum going from task to task. I thrive off feeling accomplished. I bask in the pleasure of getting things done and having everything be in its place. I like keeping my home tidy, enjoying it most when it feels perfect.

My type A, perfectionist personality was dueling with the exact opposite of everything I could understand: a type B. By nature I perform tasks at rigorous paces to satiate my achievement-driven mentality. Brandon has much lower stress levels and works at a steady pace. He enjoys achievement, but doesn't need it or crave it the way I do. I am apt to take on mountains of responsibility in my free time and he prefers to be quiet and reflective. I have a tendency to push for what I want with urgency, whereas he lives with a more accommodating and cooperative attitude toward life (and thankfully toward me as well).

The world as I knew it was punctured.

I was married to someone who shined a light on all of my perfectionistic idiosyncrasies. It was possibly the best thing to ever happen to me.

Thanks to Brandon I started to see the problem with the bubble of my perfectionism. In my pursuit of achievement and perfection, I lived with deep anxiety and constant pressure. I wanted to be and have it all. In school I wanted a scholarship, good grades, popularity, respect, and athletic success. I got all of them, fueling my drive even deeper. My high school and college years were stained by bulimia, a binge-eating disorder, and a compulsive exercise addiction in my quest to perfect my body and weight. As I started my career in the fitness industry, I quickly beat every personal training sales record, had clients with record-breaking results, and rose rapidly into management positions. I set income goals for myself and exceeded them. I tackled major athletic accomplishments and became a recognized athlete with sponsorships. It seemed like my perfectionist mind-set was making life work well for me.

The thing is, despite all of my success, there was something missing. I figured this out a few weeks after I had achieved one of my lifetime goals—crossing the finish line of an Ironman competition. Elation is the only word to describe how it felt to cross the line after swimming 2.4 miles, biking 112 miles, and running 26.2 miles. It was one of the best days of my life. But eventually the wonder faded. My heart felt empty. I felt uneasy all the time.

I had achieved everything I had ever wanted, but it didn't satisfy me. In fact, it actually incited more internal pressure to find a new high that could temporarily satisfy my yearning for accomplishment and worth. I was caught on the hamster wheel of perfectionism.

My wheel broke the day I decided to finally be honest with myself. In love with my husband and emboldened by a glass of cabernet, the question, *What am I trying to prove and to whom*, rattled around in my brain over and over until tears broke on my face. Looking up toward the heavens I had my answer. The answer could not have been clearer. My original meditative question faded in exchange for a statement: *I have nothing to prove because I am already as loved as I possibly ever could be.* In that moment, for the very first time, I experienced contentment.

The problem with perfectionism is that it separates us from any ability to find contentment. Perfectionism actually brings out the worst in us as it compels us to believe that nothing we do will ever be good enough. Driven by a need to earn approval, acceptance, and applause, perfectionists curate behaviors that drive them far from any state of peace or grace. In a constant quest to matter, perfectionists lose sight of the reason why they really matter—for who they are, not for what they do.

Like lemmings walking off a cliff, perfectionists represent a mass of society who believe the façade that being perfect is attainable, and worse than that, the lie that it is desirable. It is a never-ending cycle and the only way to break free from it is to puncture its lifeline—the lie that we need to be and do it all. The most effective way to break the complex conviction and compulsion of perfectionism is to flood yourself with truth.

The truth is that God created you and He loves you. He crafted you with intention and specification to be exactly who He wants you to be. There is nothing you can do to earn His love and there is nothing you can do to lose His love. He is for you, not against you. You are His child. His loved one. His perfect creation.

I dare you to believe this.

Do not let the word "perfectionist" be a part of your identity any longer. Cut it from you. Prune it from your personal identity. Let others know that you are no longer a perfectionist. Metaphorically enter yourself into a recovery program. As soon as you made the decision to enter recovery, you are no longer a perfectionist. You have crossed the threshold into being a recovering perfectionist, which is a powerful step of truth to take.

Finally, as you puncture perfectionism in your life you must keep your heart open to the constant reprogramming that it will undertake. Be encouraged that with every small update your heart incurs, you are moving forward. You have punctured the pattern.

PHYSICAL DETOX
Squeeze Relaxation

Perfectionism is an expression of anxiety. It is an inability to slow down and relax. In this physical detox you are going to literally put your body into a state of relaxation. This strategy will help you as you continue your recovery as a perfectionist and it is also a useful tool to employ before going to sleep at night if you struggle with worry or restlessness.

Lying down, close your eyes; take a deep breath in through your nostrils and then a long, extended breath out through your mouth. Starting with your toes, squeeze your feet together, scrunching your feet tightly in a hold for five full seconds. After the five seconds, release your feet into full re-laxation, sending your breath down through your feet and to your toes. Next, progress to your calves and leg muscles, con-tracting them as tightly as possible and holding them firmly in contraction for five full seconds. Release, sending breath and relaxation toward each leg and then move upward in your body toward your gluteus muscles. Continue this squeeze/release sequence moving upward throughout your body, making sure you perform the squeeze on every part of your body. Your final squeeze will involve your facial muscles. After you complete a squeeze on the entire body, rest in a state of calm relaxation with steady and controlled breathing for an additional two minutes.

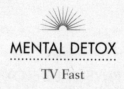

MENTAL DETOX
TV Fast

We are often seduced into perfectionism from the external in-fluences that we allow into our minds. Television—from its programs to its commercials—is one of the most common disruptors to our own state of self-satisfaction. Watching too much or the wrong kind of TV awakens restlessness, insecu-rity, and comparison within our spirits, driving us toward a mind-set of perfectionism and achievement-based worth.

Cleanse yourself for the next five days by unplugging your television set completely. Go on a television—or online TV streaming—detox. Be prepared with alternative activities such as a stack of good books, board games, or a home project to replace your normal TV watching time. The first few days will be a little tough, but by day three you should feel more at peace with the quiet in your home and the clarity in your thoughts.

SPIRITUAL DETOX

Possessing Your Position

Thank you for making me so wonderfully complex! Your workmanship is marvelous—how well I know it. (Psalm 139:14)

Perfectionism is grounded in the belief that who you are is not good enough. It is the pursuit of earning a position of worth and praise in the eyes of others. As you now know, however, your position is already determined. You are perfect as you are. You are exactly who you are meant to be. To break free of perfectionism you must possess the position that you were fearfully and wonderfully made. As other biblical translations of Psalm 139:14 state, you are "wonderfully complex" (New Living Translation), "remarkably made" (Holman Christian Standard Bible), and "body and soul, [you are] marvelously made" (The Message).

Possess this position—the perfection with which God already sees you—with confidence by utilizing the following lines to write out exactly what it is about you that is worthy of praise. Consider the miraculous way that God knit you together in your mother's womb, your unique physical traits, your personality strengths, and the character that God has breathed into your heart.

....
....
....
....
....
....
....
....

....

Father, I praise You for Your son Jesus Christ,
Who was and is perfect and Who died on the cross
for me, so that I do not need to be perfect. I give
to You my perfectionistic thinking and submit
myself to changing my focus from a pursuit of
perfection to instead a pursuit of excellence.
In the excellent name of Jesus, Amen.

FEAR

The Truth: You can fight fear by
surrounding yourself with love.

Cast out all fear with love; you will never find freedom to be who
you are meant to be if fear is present in your heart and life.

Fear Addict

A few years ago, when I started my first business, fear became
very real to me. The adventures and confidence of my youth
seemed irrelevant to the risk that comes with the venture of
becoming my own boss. The stakes were high—my business
was more than just my dream, I knew it was my calling—and
a fear of failure was so intimately entwined in my every action
that it felt like a tangible part of me. I lost sleep, I lost faith,
and I lost happiness.

It was at this time of my life that the words of Eleanor
Roosevelt became my credo.

She said, *"Do one thing every day that scares you,"* and I
took her words seriously. Additionally, her comment that *"you
must do the thing you think you cannot do"* spurred me on to

taking action on the daunting challenges that had previously cast shadows on my confidence.

I decided to live by Roosevelt's advice and started intentionally writing each scary conquest I took on through a simple tally list on my iPhone. Sometimes I tackled small fears, other times large ones. Small or large, it didn't matter; I was in training to overcome fear.

As the last few years have passed, the adventures I have taken on have been building upon themselves. It was on my honeymoon in Bora Bora that I most recently stood on the ledge, literally, and faced my fear.

My husband, Brandon, and I spent a full day on a snorkeling excursion: it was the perfect opportunity to see all of the islands and to become like fish in the gorgeous waters boasting forty-two different shades of blue. I was surprised when our tour guide brought us to water that was the darkest blue we had seen that day. He stood on the ledge of the boat, with flippers on his feet, gave an emphatic speech, and then dove backward into the clear water.

I'm not sure if it was more awe or fear that brought me to peer over the boat's edge, but I found myself staring past this crazy Tahitian guide treading in the water below. When he waved us to dive in, I hesitated. Below his kicking feet were twelve-foot lemon sharks, lots of them. Even though I know lemon sharks aren't notoriously vicious, they are still sharks. Fear makes everything bigger and they were definitely bigger than me. I was less focused on their overall size and more on their jaws, which were huge, big enough to make me their lunch. In a moment I became tiny and afraid.

At that moment Eleanor's words echoed in my mind. *"Do*

one thing every day that scares you. Do one thing every day that scares you. Do one thing every day that scares you." I knew this was my opportunity. My heart raced. And then I jumped.

The cool water refreshed my courage. The guide motioned for me to dive deeper to *touch* the sharks. I couldn't believe I was actually swimming with sharks. I watched through my goggles as he reached out and petted them as if they were nothing more than tame fish. I mustered up all my courage and dove down with my hand extended. A coarse sandpaper texture rubbed across my fingertips as I timidly brushed the shark's back. My lungs screaming for air, I swam back to the surface to catch my breath and count my fingers.

My fingers were intact and my courage swelled. I resubmerged to dive deeper.

Following the guide's lead, I grabbed on to one of the shark's fins. Like a horse under reins, the shark took off, giving me the ride of my life. I was hooked. For the next twenty minutes I chased these docile sharks. I rode on their backs as if I were surfing, I petted their giant underbellies, and I laughed at the absurdity of it all.

Life really does begin when you step outside your comfort zone. Had I never jumped off the boat ledge, had I not ignored my fear, I would have never been able to say that I have surfed a shark. Each and every time we choose to face our fear we are strengthening our inner state of love for life. We are saying "no" to fear and "yes" to a life unafraid.

I love the adventure inherent in trying new things. The ability to try new things—and to have new adventures in life—stems directly from an ability to face fear. Fear is common to everyone. Fear displays itself in many disguises by binding people to anxiety, worry, perfectionism, uncertainty, angst, dread, and general uneasiness. We can become so accustomed to fear that it can become our comfort zone. Most people will never admit to having a fear addiction, but they do. Below the surface, we are all plagued with doubts and insecurities. All insecurity comes from fear. We fear not being good enough, not being successful enough, not being beautiful enough, not being skinny enough, not being special enough, not being, well, enough. Our deep craving for acceptance drives the fear of not being accepted even deeper and more rooted into our hearts, causing the fear cycle to be placed on repeat. If we want to overcome fear we must get used to facing fear, because like anything, it takes practice. It sounds counterintuitive to seek out fear, but it is in fact the only way to ever overcome it.

The best way to do this is to step out and jump into it. The scarier the jump, the more rewarding the discovery will be. It unveils character, strength, and fortitude buried deep.

Jump off the ledge, go surf some sharks, and remember, do one thing every day that scares you.

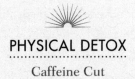

PHYSICAL DETOX
Caffeine Cut

One of the most common addictions that people battle is a caffeine addiction. Caffeine is the most widely abused drug in the world. In and of itself, caffeine is not inherently bad. Caffeine can, however, have negative effects when abused.

Caffeine has been associated with:

- Insomnia
- Feeling jittery and skittish
- Headaches
- Upset stomach from acidic effects
- Increased heart rate
- Dehydration

Cut down your caffeine and you will most likely:

- Sleep more soundly
- Experience less anxiety
- Feel more balanced
- Improve your digestive system
- Be better hydrated, leading to increased metabolism

Your physical detox today is to take on the "Caffeine Cut." Since caffeine is often associated with a higher level of anxiety—or fear—cutting down on your caffeine intake can be a tool in your fight against fear in your life.

To cut your caffeine for the sake of this detox, first assess just how much caffeine you actually consume per day. You can find a great reference guide on my website at www.trishblackwell.com/caffeinechart.

Once you have determined your average consumption, make a goal to cut your caffeine intake in half for the next five days. You may experience a slight headache on the first day or two of the detox, but stay the course. The headaches will go away and you will find yourself feeling amazing very shortly.

Caffeine can be intoxicating. Its addictive nature convinces us that we need it to ignite our energy and personality. As you cut caffeine this week, you will be able to tap into your natural energy sources. Additionally, as your energy awareness increases, you will be more in tune with your body's needs. The quality of your sleep will improve as will your ability to focus when you are awake. I would love to know how your caffeine detox goes, so please tweet me @trainerTRISH, using the hashtag #insecuritydetox after you complete day five and let me know how you feel!

MENTAL DETOX

Setting Up a Service Station

My mom taught me a great way to overcome fear. Actually, it's great for overcoming anxiety, helplessness, or any other emotional state of distraught. She told me, "Trish, when you're out of gas, set up a service station."

It works. If you feel down, overwhelmed, or fearful, the only way out is to focus on others. The idea of setting up a service station means that you commit that day to serving and loving others. Through the process of "filling their tanks," or building them up, you will help fill yours as well.

Do something today that serves others. You could surprise your coworkers with breakfast sandwiches, take a friend out to lunch, or offer to mow an elderly neighbor's lawn. Any type of service toward others will fill your heart with love. Set up a service station of your own this week and focus on how you can love others with more sincerity, more action, and more truth. As you saturate yourself in love, your heart will be filled with peace. The state of peace that you find will drive out any negativity—that is, anxiety, worry, uneasiness, or any expression of fear that might be burdening you—and you will be cleansed of a restless emotional state.

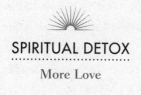

SPIRITUAL DETOX

More Love

We know how much God loves us, and we have put our trust in his love. God is love, and all who live in love live in God, and God lives in them. And as we live in God our love grows more perfect. So we will not be afraid on the day of judgment, but we can face him with confidence because we live like Jesus here in the world. Such love has no fear, because perfect love expels all fear. If we are afraid, it is for fear of punishment and this shows that we have not fully experienced his perfect love. We love each other because he loved us first. (1 John 4:16–19)

The most important thing we could ever know about our own identity is that God loves us. He loves us for who we are, not for what we do to earn His heart or affection. Love comes from God. It is who He is. The most succinct definition of God is found in the Scripture above, 1 John 4:16, "God is love." There is no better way to drive out fear than to dwell in the truth of the unconditional love that God has for us. There is nothing that we can do to make God love us more and there is nothing we can do to make God love us less. His love is unreserved, unlimited, unrestricted, unmitigated, and unquestioning. We are loved because He loves us. There is no arguing with the love of God. If He says we are lovable, then we are. If He says we are accepted and perfect in Him, then we are. In the love of God, this magnificent love, there is freedom.

You can be free from fear because you have the love of God within you. Your spiritual detox today is to love more. Find three ways to actively express love today in the following categories. It is impossible to exhaust your heart of love when you are plugged into the love of God, so let your love flow. You are empowered to let love reign—and thereby the peace that comes with love—as you face every fear that comes your way. You can write in your ideas below:

How I can love myself more:

....

....

....

How I can love my family and friends more:

....

....

....

How I can love God more:

....

....

....

....

Father, thank You for Your perfect love that casts out all fear. I give to You all of my fears and I trust that no matter what happens, You are in control and Your love will always win over the darkness I fear. Teach me to fight fear boldly. Pour over my heart more love than I could ever imagine possible. In the fearless name of Jesus, Amen.

NEGATIVITY

The Truth: You are allergic to negativity.

You can start a personal war on negativity by avoiding it like
you would avoid something you are allergic to.

Watercooler Gossip

Recently, I learned that I have an allergy to dill. To my misfortune, I also discovered that I love dill. Being the extremist that I am, when I love something, I really love hard. I ravaged my local farmers' market, buying bouquets of it at a time to create dill salads that I devoured. Then something terrible happened. Shortly into this gastronomical love affair I discovered that dill did not love me back. I woke one morning to hives covering my entire body. They were painful, itchy, and everywhere. It was a sad day. I threw the rest of my dill out, went to the doctor, and waited two weeks for my body to heal.

A few months later I convinced myself that just a little bit of dill wouldn't do me any harm. Attributing my hive outbreak to the sheer quantity of dill I consumed, I decided to reintroduce dill back into my life in a small quantity. I indulged by dipping some broccoli in a dill-based vegetable dip. Dill is dill though, and unfortunately a little bit affected me just as much as a lot does.

Negativity is a lot like my dill allergy. It only takes a little exposure of negativity to feel its damaging effect on our minds. Even though I am a naturally positive and optimistic person, I wasted years of my life not protecting myself from the negativity of people around me. Without realizing it, I internalized the by-product toxins of negativity and ended up with a battlefield in my mind. Fundamentally I was positive, but practically I was bombarded with self-doubt, self-criticism, and self-limiting thoughts.

We've all been there; it's a conversation that sucks you in too easily. You don't like it but you stay engaged. You might be at the watercooler, out on the town with some friends, at the grocery store, or just in the locker room at the gym—these conversations pop up everywhere.

You walk away from the exchange feeling off but you can't put your finger on exactly why or what went wrong.

You are having an allergic reaction. It is an allergic reaction to negativity.

The negativity wasn't obvious. The conversations seemed innocuous, but they weren't and they aren't. Gossip is like that. It starts innocently and morphs subliminally into something toxic. Small talk can be similar. What starts as small talk develops into complaining, self-bashing, and a general discussion of discontent about the mundane details of life.

Whether we realize it or not, this is one allergy we all have. Unfortunately, unlike a food allergy, we can't simply choose not to ingest it because we are inundated daily with influences that force the allergy on us. Since negativity—cynics, critics, complainers, gossips, bad-news bearers, self-promoters, drama queens, pessimists, and those with a victim mentality—surrounds us, we need to live on guard and be prepared to fight back.

We have available to us a metaphorical EpiPen. It is an evacuation button and works as quickly as an autoinjection of epinephrine does for someone who is experiencing an intense allergic reaction to a substance or food. This EpiPen is your ability to walk away. It is your ability to choose your thoughts. It is your discernment in the company with which you surround yourself and the content you allow to enter your mind. It is your knowledge that what you feed in your life is what will grow, and so you feed positivity and you starve negativity.

We must starve the negativity in our lives. The more we give into self-doubt, complaining, and fear, the more we are feeding those thoughts in our minds, making them more prominent and ingrained. To break the cycle—and to feed positivity—we must be proactively aware. We must realize that even a little bit of negativity can have toxic measures on our lives. In the same way that I can't eat dill anymore because the side effects of just a little are as noxious as a lot, so, too, is a little negativity as dangerous as a lot. To starve negativity we must be cognizant of the ways that it seeps into our lives.

Starve the negativity allergens in your life by choosing to:

- Walk away from negative conversations.
- Minimize the amount of news and media gossip you allow to capture your attention.
- Choose your friends wisely
- Spend more time with optimists.
- Capture your self-critical thoughts and reposition them with truth about who you are.

- Refuse to engage in gossip—and know that even listening to gossip is participating in it.
- Saturate your mind with truth and with anything that speaks positively to your potential.
- Surround yourself with uplifting resources— people, books, music, podcasts, and experiences.
- Be a stickler for choosing the right attitude no matter what circumstances come your way.
- Become known as someone who is allergic to negativity and avoids it like the plague.

PHYSICAL DETOX

Epsom Salt Bath

As you purge yourself from exposure to negativity in your life, prepare to purge your body from toxins that have built up internally. By taking an Epsom salt bath, you have the opportunity to relax your mind and spirit at the same time you are actually detoxing your body.

Epsom salt can be found at any local pharmacy or grocery store and is not actually salt, but rather a pure mineral compound of magnesium and sulfate. The magnesium in the Epsom salt regulates your natural enzymes, reduces inflammation, improves muscle function, and reduces artery inflammation. The sulfate component of the soaking compound flushes toxins from the body naturally as well as increases the skin's ability to absorb nutrients.

To maximize this physical detox, purchase a few bags of

Epsom salt (you can get them without scent, or with a lavender or eucalyptus scent) and set aside thirty minutes to relax. Run warm water, light some candles in your bathroom, and slowly pour Epsom salt into your warm bath water. Once you get in you will notice some of the salt crystals around you, but after a few minutes these crystals will dissolve and be absorbed naturally through your skin. Do your best to submerge yourself in the water so every part of your body can benefit from the cleansing power of the Epsom salt.

MENTAL DETOX
Pattern Interruption

Avoiding negativity in your life is going to take effort and discipline. In many ways it will demand that you engage in pattern interruption—that is, a disruption of your current daily habits. To strengthen you for this change of behavior, your mental detox activity is to practice a variety of mundane pattern interruptions in your life. The more used to pattern interruption you are, the more flexible and open you will become, preparing you to be successful at disrupting the negative patterns and influences in your life.

To practice pattern interruption, try the following suggestions and activities:

- Choose a new route to work, even if it takes longer.
- Change up your evening routine by not turning on the TV for a week.
- Turn off your social media notifications and only

permit yourself to engage in social media once a
day instead of multiple times throughout the day.

- Eat with your nondominant hand . . . if you are
  right-handed and normally use a fork in your
  right hand, practice eating a few meals with the
  fork in your left hand.
- Forgo your morning coffee two days in a row.
- Order something different at your favorite restaurant or make a meal at home that you haven't
  made in months.

SPIRITUAL DETOX

Forgiveness Letter

But when you are praying, first forgive anyone you are holding a grudge against,
so that your Father in heaven will forgive your sins too. (Mark 11:25)

Unforgiveness is a burden that can hold us captive to a negative spirit. In order to really cleanse yourself from negativity—
and to continue to minimize its presence in your life—you
must find freedom in forgiveness. Forgive yourself for the flaws
of your past that you keep rehashing, forgive others for the
wrong they have done to you, and be forgiven of all your sins
by accepting Jesus Christ as your Lord and Savior.

Forgiveness gives us freedom. A lack of forgiveness binds
us to chains and keeps us locked inside a prison of darkness
and negativity.

If you are holding a grudge or holding on to pain someone

caused you—or perhaps that you even caused yourself—write a short letter of forgiveness. In your letter include how they made you feel, how you forgive them or want to forgive them, and then ask God to give you the strength to make that happen. Send the letter if you'd like, but burn it (after forgiving the person) if you don't send it. The act of writing the letter and then sending it off with grace—either literally or metaphorically—will cleanse your spirit and open wide the windows of freedom.

....

Father, I commit to You my thoughts. Forgive
me my negativity and my doubt, and replace
any negative tendencies I might have with a
confident approach seeped in faith and trust in
You. In the positive name of Jesus, Amen.

LACK OF CONFIDENCE

The Truth: You are who you are meant to be.

The key in learning how to be confident is embracing who He made you to be instead of striving to fit the mold of others' expectations.

Genie-Pants Power

Brandon has a pair of green lounge pants that are absolutely hideous and three sizes too big. He refuses to throw them away. Reminiscent of MC Hammer pants, they could also stand in as genie pants. Simply put, they are ridiculous. Every now and then he embarrasses me by wearing them outside the house when he mows the lawn.

Even though I've had the opportunity, and desperately want to, I am unable to bring myself to throw them away because he wears those pants with confidence. There is something attractive about Brandon's goofy attachment to these pants. He wears them with swagger. In a weird way, they reflect his individuality and his determination to never sway from being himself, even though I have told him over and over just how ridiculous they look on him.

I have swayed from being myself far too many times. The pressure of other peoples' opinions has weighed on me and persuaded me to try to be someone other than my true self. As a result I spent years of my life as a social chameleon, trying to blend in with my surroundings. I questioned the clothes I wore, felt insecure about how I styled my hair, and was constantly adapting my personality to blend in with whichever group of friends I was around. Living this way is exhausting and lonely. It's hard to feel authentically connected to anyone if you aren't even able to connect to yourself.

I finally learned to simply embrace being myself, and only myself, after I graduated from college. Thanks to my two wonderful friends Caroline and Angi, with whom I spent a year in France, I started to get a taste of what it feels like to be free to be me. Together the three of us "worked" as English teachers and spent as much time as we could playing hooky from work in order to gallivant through the French countryside as much as we could. Caroline and Angi were beautiful, quirky, and committed to being unapologetically themselves in a foreign country. Angi—an actress—takes the world as her stage and is apt to take any opportunity to perform in public. Caroline was guided by goofiness and clowned around with children, animals, and strangers alike. In a country of structure and pomp these two girls burst open the seams of expectations. Their example was so intoxicating that it was impossible to resist imitating. Imitation didn't lead to mimicry, but rather inspired me to embrace my quirks and live without fear of being myself. When a social chameleon joins a group of people who are free to be themselves, she is forced to try to do the same.

Too many of us waste years of our lives trying to be someone we are not. We drive ourselves mad trying to imitate the
people we want to be. Mimicking their lifestyle, we prescribe
ourselves a destiny that was determined for someone else and
wonder why our plans don't quite work out as we expected.
And while it's okay to emulate someone we look up to, it's entirely different to try to live out *their* stories instead of our own.

Don't underestimate the power of being unique. Being
unique means that you have something to offer the rest of the
world that no one else does. My time in France awakened me
to this truth, but it wasn't until later that it was reinforced and
ingrained into my soul. My boss at the time, Kim, repeated one
phrase over and over to me, upwards of two hundred times:

"There's only one Trish Blackwell."

I would smile, thank her for her kind words, and casually
shrug off the compliment. Sensing my disbelief, she would insist
again. *"Blackwell, I'm serious. There's only one Trish Blackwell."*

It was hard to hear and even harder to believe, but eventually, thanks to the repetition of her words and her insis-
tence, I started to believe her. She continued this exercise for
months, often requiring me to look directly at myself in the
mirror and repeat the phrase *"There's only one Trish Blackwell"*
out loud to myself. After the words became more natural for
me to hear and say she added more words of life. *"There's only
one Trish Blackwell, and she has tons of potential to do great
things in the world with how God created her to be."*

After enough repetition and persistence on her part, I
started to see myself differently. I started to finally see what
God saw in me. I started to learn to love myself. I started to
see that I was unique and that God had breathed into me a
story to live out and share with the world.

Confidence is an inside job. The more we embrace our one-of-a-kind identity—even if it includes genie pants—the more confident we will feel. The more we believe and accept ourselves for the masterpieces we were created to be, the more alive we will feel. The ability to be ourselves freely—quirks and all—can elevate our confidence to new levels, freeing us in how we live our daily lives.

You are one of one. I know this sounds simple, but it is actually astoundingly complex. Just think about the fact that there is no one who has the same fingerprints, taste buds, personality traits, voice, or genetic makeup as you. It's time to start seeing yourself for just how priceless you are. Like a masterpiece of artwork, you are unable to be replicated, and you are therefore invaluable. Expending your time and energy being a copy of anyone else is not only a waste of time, but also an insult to the Artist who created you. Replicas of great artwork are never as good or as valuable as the original piece anyway, so stay true to your original self and to the person God created and crafted you to be.

PHYSICAL DETOX

Assess Your Wardrobe

We all have a pair of green genie pants—a beloved item of clothing that is just ridiculous. You might feel like you should toss it, but don't. Keep it if it makes you happy, even if it is too big, too small, ugly, or out of style. Loving the clothes that you wear—for whatever reason you love them—will help you feel more confident. When you feel confident you will walk around with confidence; when you walk around with confidence you will be confident.

Detox your wardrobe of anything that you own that doesn't make you feel amazing about your body. As you sort through your clothes, make a pile of clothes that don't fit well and set them aside to donate to charity. Make a separate pile for clothes like Brandon's green genie pants—clothes that truly make you happy—and be sure to keep those. If you find that you don't have enough clothes that flatter your figure, then it's time to splurge on a shopping spree for yourself. Everyone deserves to wear clothes that make them happy and that fit them well.

MENTAL DETOX
Year List

Embrace your individuality by creating a list of individual goals for yourself to accomplish this year. This mental detox is your "Five for the Year" list and represents the pursuit of what makes you the person you are. Create your list by first thinking about the top five interests that currently captivate your heart. Take those interests and carve a specific goal out of each one, using the space below to write them down.

My Five for the Year:

1) ....

2) ....

3) ....

4) ....

5) ....

Finally, once you have determined your Five for the Year, select *one word* that will summarize and define the rest of the year for you. This word should be a positive and powerful word and you can use it as a mental mantra for yourself to fuel you forward as you work toward your Five for the Year. Use the space below to proclaim your Word for the Year:

My Word for the Year:

....

SPIRITUAL DETOX

The Laughter Medicine

We were filled with laughter, and we sang for joy. And the other nations said, "What amazing things the Lord has done for them." (Psalm 126:2)

The most confidence-inspiring thing I learned from my friendship with Caroline and Angi was the power of laughter, and in particular, the power of having the ability to laugh at myself. Laughter is one of the most effective ways to break down any invisible walls of insecurity that hold us back from embracing our full unique personality. When we laugh we are free. The more you laugh the easier it becomes to laugh. Laughter is contagious and it teaches our souls to see the world with a sunny and confident disposition.

Be free to be yourself by incorporating more laughter into your life. Find a way to laugh today, either by making an effort to be around a funny friend, watching a comedy show or movie, or reading a funny book. Laughter is a shining expression of the soul at the core of how God made us. God loves it when His children laugh; we were made to enjoy life and to enjoy Him.

Laughter is a dose of medicine that releases your inner self to be free and quirky. It is one of the most beautiful sounds we can elicit. Your spiritual detox today is to spend ten minutes intentionally investing in laughter. Take this detox to the next level by repeating the challenge for five days in a row. Here are some suggestions to incorporate these ten minutes of laughter into your day:

Laugh more by:

- Smiling at yourself in the mirror and acting out a laugh; even though the laugh isn't natural it will evoke and inspire natural laughter to come.
- Watching a funny TV show or movie—know your sense of humor to know what kind of program to watch that will elicit a good laugh from yourself.
- Reading a comic strip online.
- Tickling someone.
- Giving yourself permission to play . . . play pretend with a kid you know.
- Hanging out with people who have a sense of humor.
- Watching someone else laugh.

- Laughing at yourself about something silly you've done in the past.

....

Father, I am confident in who You created me to be. Show me how I can choose to cling to this godly confidence every day as I walk the path You have set out before me. Give me unwavering faith that I am who I need to be because I was created masterfully in Your image. In the masterful name of Jesus, Amen.

SMALL DREAMS

*The Truth: You have permission to
dream big and do big things.*

*The dreams we dream are too small in proportion to the
greatness and the life that God has placed within us.*

Cascading Expectations

The day my brother tried to dig up dinosaur bones in our back-yard was the first time my parents realized that he had a passion for excavation. When dinosaur bones weren't to be found, he decided to dig for Noah's Ark. He didn't find Noah's Ark, but eventually he stumbled upon some Civil War relics from the Battle of the Wilderness of 1864. The Civil War literally took place in our backyard. Nick was hooked. He had high expectations of what he could discover, and he held strongly to those convictions. Nick's interest peaked more and more over the years, eventually leading him to a PhD in classical Greek studies, making him an archaeologist. He and his family live abroad and travel the world, bouncing between exotic archaeological destinations and studies.

I am no archaeologist, but I do share a similar passion for exploration. And while my husband, Brandon, and I list international travel as our favorite way to explore, we believe exploration is a mind-set and can be engaged wherever we are. Together we explore local restaurants, vineyards, artisan shops, local towns, and National Parks.

Recently we went for a hike in Shenandoah National Park. I expertly navigated us to the base entrance of what I thought was Old Rag Mountain. It turns out that we weren't at Old Rag, but we did land at a National Park entrance where the park ranger promised us a hike decorated with waterfalls. I am a sucker for waterfalls, so I was in and Brandon was, too.

Excitedly, we ventured along the narrow, serpentine trail that followed a rocky stream. The ranger had told us that we would encounter seven magnificent waterfalls and I was prepared to have my breath taken away from me.

After a few miles there were no dramatic waterfalls to be found. Slightly disappointed I still held on to my hopes of majestic cascades. The hike started to drag; the lack of scenery change and waterfalls made me reset my expectations. With no waterfalls in sight, I resigned myself to believe that the small rapids in the rocky stream must have been the referenced waterfalls. Saddened by the outcome of the so-called falls, I rallied by settling for a smaller vision of what I expected. I made peace with the beauty of what surrounded us and we continued along our merry way, soaking up the sunshine with gratitude. I acquiesced to these new lower expectations and re-framed what I considered to be a waterfall.

And then the path took a turn.

Without warning, our rocky trail opened up to an eighty-three-foot double waterfall. The unexpected grandeur of it all was so breathtaking it stopped me dead in my tracks. After that point, we were greeted with a parade of impressive falls, to such an extent that I wondered why I ever was willing to change my standard in the first place.

The park ranger had not let us down. The waterfalls he spoke of were truly magnificent, and furthermore, the length of time it took to arrive at their base made them all the more marvelous. There are things in life that cannot be rushed, and arriving at a promised waterfall is one of them.

The way we see ourselves is often similar to the waterfalls from my hike. We are told that there is something great and majestic within us—placed and purposed by God Himself—yet we lower and settle our expectations based upon what we have seen thus far. We know that the promise of greatness is within us, but we weary along the path and we lose hope. Somewhere along the way we learn to compromise, somewhere we believe the lie that we are just average, and somewhere we redefine our identities, selling ourselves short in the same way I dared compare a small rapid to a magnificent waterfall.

In the heart of every human being lies a desire to discover his or her destiny. We want to know that we matter. We want to know that we are loved. We want to know that we can really live and make a difference in this world. The exploration of these three desires—to live, to love, and to matter—is what equips us to live with confident anticipation toward life. We get tied up, however, when the promise of possibility seems too far off or out of reach for us to actually experience. And that is when we begin to sell ourselves short. That is when we lose confidence and we start calling a rapid a waterfall.

You have to believe in the waterfalls that are to come, even when all you can see are rapids.

Even though Nick didn't discover Noah's Ark, he never lowered his expectations on what he could and would find. We must not lower our expectations because by doing so we remove ourselves from a position of potential. To fulfill your potential you must get up and travel your path. Keep walking, even if the path is serpentine and feels like the waterfalls you have envisioned might never arrive, because you never know what you will run into when you turn the next corner. The only way to discover the waterfalls is to keep walking and keep exploring. The only way to live out the dream that has been sown into your heart is to believe that it is there and to live in daily pursuit of it, never lowering your expectations and never doubting the greatness that has been breathed into you by God Himself.

PHYSICAL DETOX

Stress Less, Move More

Stress inhibits the potential of our lives, often convincing us to dream smaller dreams than we have within us. As I said earlier, stress is an often underestimated factor with a major impact on our physical and mental health. When stress occurs, the body releases a hormone called cortisol, which sends a message to the body to store fat, particularly around the stomach region. Stress can literally keep you from achieving and maintaining your ideal body weight.

One of the most effective ways to relieve stress is to move

your body more. This doesn't always have to be in the format of a structured workout; you just have to be more active in general. Physical exertion is correlated with stress relief and release. Furthermore, the more you move your body, the more natural dopamine will be released, giving you an endorphin-induced energy that will energize you physically and mentally.

Below are some tips on practical ways to stress less and move more that won't demand more from your schedule:

Stress Less

- Prioritize sleep.
- Talk to someone you trust about your problems.
- Give your mind a break.
- Create a daily to-do list with three main priorities for the day.
- Ask for help from others when you need it.
- Remember that you are not expected to be perfect.
- Start saying "no" to overloading your schedule.
- Drink herbal tea at night.
- Take a bath.
- Self-massage.

Move More

- Pick a parking spot that is the farthest in the lot from your destination.
- Go for a walk after lunch and dinner.
- Stretch for three minutes when you first wake up.
- Find an exercise buddy and schedule a workout date with them.

- Put your workouts in your calendar as if they were important meetings—with a high priority and as non-negotiable.

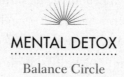

MENTAL DETOX
....
Balance Circle

It is easy to have misaligned expectations when your life feels out of balance. When life feels out of balance we are less apt to pursue the giant dreams and great expectations that have been placed in our hearts.

Take just five minutes to self-assess the balance of all elements of your life by using the "Circle of Balance" on the next page. For each category, give yourself an honest assessment on a scale of 1 to 10 for how strong and focused you feel in your life for that particular category. A rating of a 10 means that you spend a lot of time, energy, and focus on that category and feel confident that you are well invested in it; a rating of a 0 means that you don't spend any time or effort on that category.

Once you assess your rating for each category, mark it with a dot on the corresponding diagram. After you have graded yourself and dotted all ten categories, take a pen and connect the dots to form a circle.

The goal of this exercise is to assess the balance of your circle, not necessarily to score high in all categories. So, for example, if you have a rating of 7 to 9 on 6 of your categories, but then score a 2 to 4 on the remaining 2, you will end up with a very lopsided wheel or circle. In such a scenario, your growth goal would be to focus on the two categories where you scored low, attempting to spend more time on them to bring them to balance with your other scores of 7, 8, and 9. In order to do so you may have to remove some of the attention that you spend on your 8 and 9 categories so as to have time to equalize your growth in your weaker categories.

Once you live with a balanced "wheel" for all ten categories, you will have a more balanced perspective and be able to manage and align your expectations of life more positively and appropriately.

THE CIRCLE OF BALANCE

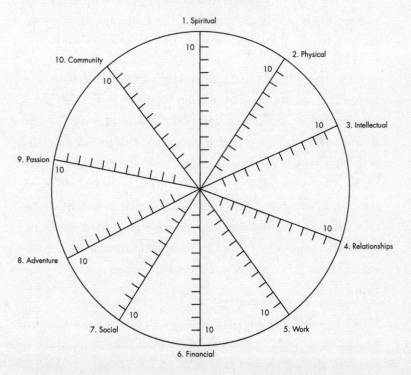

* A special thanks to my mentor Todd Durkin for introducing me to the concept of assessing my overall balance in life with the tool of a self-assessment circle.

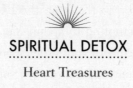

SPIRITUAL DETOX

Heart Treasures

Wherever your treasure is, there the desires of your heart will also be. (Matthew 6:21)

Where your heart is, there your treasure will also be. In order to dream—and pursue with high and confident expectation—the dream that God has placed in your heart, you must first know what you love and what you treasure in your heart. We are each gifted with different interests—different things that make our souls sing. By pursuing these unique passions we are able to unveil the true treasure that is buried in our heart.

Use the space below to dig deep into why you love what you love. Pick two things that absolutely make your heart sing. These are your heart treasures. Next, shovel out exactly what it is about these things that you love. Do this by asking yourself *"Why* do I really love or enjoy this?" and then ask *"Why"* again. Allow yourself to get as descriptive as possible to paint the beauty of what draws your heart to that love. This exercise will help you identify and excavate even more meaning and ownership out of these loves by helping you to identify exactly what it is about these loves that brings a song to your heart.

Heart Treasure #1: ....

....

....

....

....

....

Heart Treasure #2:   ....

....

....

....

....

....

....

*Father, I turn over to You my small thinking
and my small dreams. I am ready to get off of
the sidelines of life and to engage fully in the
life You have called me to live. Embolden me
with courage and faith as I pursue living out
the abundant life You have envisioned for me.
In the abundant name of Jesus, Amen.*

THE MARKED PATH

The Truth: God works all things for your good.

We aren't responsible for paving our own paths. We are simply asked to follow Him, and He will guide us to places of beauty and life we never imagined possible.

Baby Bear Tracks

I am a sucker for baby animals. I'll gingerly follow a bunny or a chipmunk whenever I see one, and I am absolutely helpless around puppies or kittens. I always thought I would become a veterinarian until I discovered that I don't like blood or science. YouTube videos of baby animals make me giggle uncontrollably. It doesn't matter what type of animal it is, all animal babies are cute and I was made to love them.

The state of Virginia is home to a large population of black bears. Though the bears are known to be shy and secretive, they are intimidatingly large and threatening. You never want to run into a bear in the woods. They are faster than us, not to mention bigger and hungrier. The baby bears, however, are just plain adorable.

I've been lucky enough to run into a few baby bears recently while hiking. Brandon has trained me well to remember that where there is a baby bear, there is a momma bear somewhere close by, which helps me resist the urge to run after them for a snuggle.

Most recently, I saw a little snuggly guy stumbling up the side of the wooded mountains, noisily rustling piles of leaves as he sauntered a few hundred yards away from me. Meandering around, he pawed at a few tree stumps, looked directly at me, and continued exploring the sights and smells of the leaf-covered hill. I watched in pure joy, soaking up his cuteness. Moments later I spotted his momma, who had blended in with the trees and browned foliage not even twenty-five feet ahead of him on the path.

It is no wonder that I didn't see her at first. A momma bear knows the woods well. She walks calmly, barely making a sound. She knows how to be a bear. Her baby, while he has the same gifts as she, is still learning how to use those gifts. He doesn't yet know how to daintily walk through leaves, how to go unnoticed, or how to climb. He follows his momma around, and, through observation and repetition, learns. He practices using his gifts by imitating what he is being shown by someone he trusts, someone who has his best interest at heart.

The momma bear did see me; she's aware of everything happening around her baby. She looked right at me from a distance and froze her stare into my still body. I don't speak bear, but she made it clear to me to stay away. Her baby's best interest was her best interest, and if I had moved, I would have been a threat to both.

There is Someone Who has your best interest at heart. He

knew you before you were born (Psalm 139:13) and He wants
for you a hope and a future (Jeremiah 29:11). You have been
created with intention and you are being matured, in the same
way the baby bear is being cared for by his momma. In the
same way she protected her little one, so, too, does God protect you. In this, God is like us, He cherishes His children
and protects them. Guard this truth in your heart.

To grow in the gifts we have been given and to mature
into being all that we were created to be, we must follow our
Maker. We must simply step forward and follow the un-
marked path with faith. In the same way that a baby bear—or
animal of any type for that matter—stumbles when it first
learns to walk, the steps that we take toward our pursuit of
our potential won't always be stable or predictable. Most of
the time we won't even be able to see the path we are following. We will fall. We will find ourselves trying to climb trees
before we are ready and we will tumble to the ground. We
will fear the unknown of winters to come, wondering how we
will ever learn to hibernate or if we will have enough food. All
of these things will be taught, only by moving forward, little
step by little step, as we need to learn them. This is faith—
taking the next step and then the next one with full confidence that our potential is worth pursuing and that our
Maker is ahead of us on the path to guide, protect, and encourage us along the way.

There is something magical about taking on the faith of a
child—or a baby bear—and just trusting the journey that we
are on. We don't need to know every step that needs to be
taken to get us to a destination; we just need to take the next
step, and then the next one, and then the next one. There will
be times when stepping forward is difficult—the path may be

too dark, we may be injured, or we may be questioning our progress—but keep your eye on your Father ahead of you and you will never step wrong.

Be assured, you are not on this journey alone, in the same way that any little baby bear does not wander the woods alone. You may not always be able to see the momma bear behind the trees, and you may not always understand where God is, but, without fail, they are both always present. Be confident, God is watching over you; so pursue excellence in every small step you take, knowing that He is guiding you along with your best interest at heart.

PHYSICAL DETOX
Morning Transformation

Studies show that people who wake up early are more productive and effective throughout the day. If you are serious about the development of your potential you need to be serious about maximizing your mornings.

The good news is that you don't necessarily need to be a morning person in order to learn to enjoy and utilize your mornings; you just need to start making small shifts and adjustments in your sleep schedule. Even just twenty minutes of extra "you" time in the morning can make a significant difference in your life and in setting yourself up for success on any given day. Once you decide what your morning routine will be, put it in your calendar and have it scheduled. Set your clothes, coffee, and other morning needs out the night before so that there is no excuse for you to dillydally and waste precious morning time that could be spent on "you" time. Here are some suggestions of ways to maximize your mornings:

- *20 Minutes of "You" Time*: Stretch for 5 minutes, have a quiet time to pray or meditate for 5 minutes, and read for 10 minutes.

- *40 Minutes of "You" Time*: Stretch for 5 minutes, have a quiet time for prayer or meditation for 5 minutes, read for 10 minutes, and exercise for 20 minutes.

- *60 Minutes of "You" Time*: Stretch for 5 minutes, have a quiet time for prayer or meditation for 5 minutes, read for 20 minutes, and exercise for 30 minutes.

- *90 Minutes of "You" Time*: Stretch for 5 minutes, have a quiet time for prayer or meditation for 5 minutes, read for 20 minutes, and exercise for 60 minutes.

MENTAL DETOX
Quiet Study

Go someplace quiet, ideally someplace outside and in nature. Make sure you have fifteen to twenty minutes, a pen and notebook, and no agenda. Find somewhere comfortable to sit and close your eyes for two minutes. Make sure your breathing is deep and calm and allow yourself to find a full state of relaxation, focusing on just being present in the moment and clearing your mind completely. After two minutes open your eyes, open up your notebook, and record everything you hear by writing it down.

This exercise is meant to increase your awareness and thereby will increase your ability to appreciate your surroundings. The more attune we are with what is around us, the more connected we will feel to our paths of growth as we journey onward.

SPIRITUAL DETOX
Shadow Love Game

Dear friends, let us continue to love one another, for love comes from God. Anyone who loves is a child of God and knows God. (1 John 4:7)

Imagine going on a walk as a kid with your parents. The sun is behind you and is casting elongated shadows in front of you as you walk. Stretching from your feet outward, your shadow appears huge. It is long, skinny, and keeps moving as you move. The shadows to either side of you—your parents' shadows—are different. They are even bigger. Those shadows envelop yours like a hedge of protection. The shadows seem to be walking hand in hand; all three of you, and you are safe, happy, and loved.

In a similar way, your life casts a shadow. Everything you do—every person you love, every small act of kindness you perform, and every kind word you say—shines a light, thereby casting a shadow. It is a shadow that makes a difference; it is a shadow warm with love. This shadow that you are able to make is only possible because of the shadow that comes from your Heavenly Father. Just as He has surrounded your life—what you can see before you—in shadows of goodness, hope, and love, so, too, can you project a replication of that shadow onto others who cross your path.

Stretch out your shadow in your mind and fill it with love that overflows. Imagine the love that you have within being so big that it casts out before you a net of love to everyone with whom you interact. Let everyone who comes into your presence be enveloped in your love, and never forget that the love you have learned to share came from the shadow of love that was first cast upon you. This is the deployment of our potential; that we might love others more fully. Those who pursue their potential unlock their purpose, and undoubtedly, purpose always has a positive impact on others.

....

Father, I praise You for showing me that Your plan for my life is unique. Thank You for the beautiful way in which You use everything in my past for good and how, even though I may have strayed from the path You have set out for me, that You always welcome me back. In the welcoming name of Jesus, Amen.

NEGATIVE BODY IMAGE

The Truth: You are enough.

*Body confidence comes from the decision to embrace and
celebrate the skin you're in, as you are today.*

Loving the Skin You're In

My bookshelf is littered with journals. Gratitude journals.
Memory journals. Love letter journals. Dream journals. Blank
journals ready to be inked. It's no secret that I love journaling.
There has been one journal, however, that didn't just change
me, it transformed my life, and that was my word journal.

I actually had multiple word journals—one for English vocabulary words, one for French, one for Spanish, one for Ital-
ian, and at one point I even had one for Mandarin Chinese.
The pages of these journals were filled with vocabulary and
colloquialisms I picked up—mostly from the dictionaries I
carried with me—as I sharpened my lexis in the languages. As
a lexophile, I was fascinated at the power words can have in
connecting people on a more profound level.

Unfortunately, even though I knew the power of words relative to the world and the relationships around me, I didn't understand their power in my own mind.

Because of the misuse of the internal vocabulary I used toward myself, I battled insecurity and negative body-image issues for nearly a decade. My mind was an expressway of self-criticism with thoughts of negativity and judgment that came so quickly to the forefront of my mind that I didn't know there was any other way to live or think. Finding flaws with my body and my physical appearance was so natural to me that it became my way of life. I didn't hate my body, but I didn't love it. In fact, I actually felt removed from it. This detachment made me feel like a stranger in my own skin. I was suffocated and trapped underneath the layered highways of self-judgment that I had constructed without realizing it.

Curiously, the cure for a negative lifestyle existed at a café halfway around the world.

As a full-time elementary school teacher to French children, I actually only worked in a part-time capacity. In a classic example of French work-life balance, I often worked less than eight hours in a week but was paid for forty. This lifestyle presented me with more free time than I had ever had in my entire adult life. As a result, I spent hours—days even—at cafés, soaking up the culture, the coffee, and the carefree attitude of the French. It was at one of those café tables that I had an epiphany that changed my life.

My French-English dictionary open, I sat at small, round aluminum table at Le Café de la Place. The table had just enough room for the dictionary, my word journal, and the stem of my glass of Bordeaux. This particular café overlooked a plaza with fountains that brought the locals to mingle outside on beautiful days. It was the perfect people-watching spot.

I filled the pages of my word journal by looking around and absorbing every detail of life that unfolded before my café table. If I couldn't describe a particular scene in detail I would search for the words to do so with the goal of deepening the breadth of my vocabulary every day. Then one day something hit me. I couldn't describe French women well. They had the ever talked about *je ne sais quoi*, but I wanted to put a word to it and couldn't. I was magnetized and in admiration of the quintessential French woman, whom I found didn't actually fit any describable or specific stereotype. The women I observed were all beautiful and so very French, but they all had different body types, fashion styles, and personalities. I couldn't pinpoint what it was about them that so drew me in. And then that day it occurred to me: they were confident. And that is what I decided I wanted for myself.

Feeling foolish that I didn't know the French word for "confident," I hurriedly flipped through the pages of my dictionary. What I came across changed everything I knew about confidence and changed the way I saw beauty.

There is no word in French for "confident." Instead, when describing someone who has confidence there is a saying: *être bien dans sa peau,* to be well in your skin.

Well in my skin. That was exactly what I was not and what I had searched to be for ten years. The most revelatory thing about this phrase was that it applied so well to the hundreds of French women I had seen and met . . . all women whose bodies didn't necessarily fit my preconceived and critical idealization of what beauty really was.

Thus started a journey of exploration and investigation

into exactly what it means to be well in my skin. I started by carefully studying the comportment and characteristics of the French women I knew and worked with and created a list of attributes these women had learned culturally that somehow I had not.

Learning how to love the skin you're in really does change how you feel. It forces you to accept the present. It frees you from the burden of "not _____ enough" and it gives you permission to simply be yourself.

In the same way that Rome was not built in a day, my personal transformation of confidence did not happen overnight, and yours won't either. Instead, it will be a process, an ongoing one. As I emulated the example of the French women around me, I learned how to be more present in the present and thereby more connected to myself. By following this process and being patient with the unfurling of my confidence, I learned how to be myself again. There were seven main lifestyle and mind-set secrets that I picked up from the French, which cumulatively carried me to a place where, for the first time in my adult life, I felt well in the skin I was in. These seven secrets are all things that you can do today, right now, starting with this present moment:

1. *Embrace your body in the present.* Love it for how it is today, not for how you hope for it to be tomorrow.

2. *Focus on good posture.* Proper posture not only increases the natural flow of oxygen through the body, but also conveys a message of confidence to others; in

turn, as you exude confidence, people will treat you accordingly, reaffirming and strengthening the confidence you are already feeling.

3. *Never **apologize for your physical self or for what you are eating.*** Indulge in *les petits plaisirs* of life in balance—there is no need to justify anything you eat. Furthermore, never dismiss your body in conversation with others . . . making excuses of any kind (blaming weight gain on the holidays, etc.) only affirms insecurity about your body.

4. *Don't engage in diet talk with others.* Diet talk is toxic and full of negativity directed toward dissatisfaction with one's body. The French don't believe in being critical of their body because that would remove them from their ability to be happy and joyful in the present. The French do diet, but they don't talk about it or bully and pressure others into joining them. Instead, they simply substitute out a few unhealthy foods for healthier choices and make an effort to be more active.

5. *Honor your body.* Never use a workout as punishment for an indulgence. Give your body rest and the proper amount of sleep. Revel in the detail of God's workmanship in you by seeing your body as a temple.

6. *Be aware.* Be present with your body by stretching daily and through slow, deep breathing exercises to feel more connected to your body. The more aware and present you are, the better and more honorable/balanced food choices you will make, making it easier

to eat well. Ultimately your good nutrition will enable you to have a body that gets set at its perfect, natural body weight on its own.

7. ***Smile more.*** The power of a smile is intoxicating and contagious; it is also scientifically shown to make someone more attractive . . . the more attractive you feel, the more confident you will be about your body.

Loving the skin you are in starts with a simple decision to start loving yourself today. Your body does not need to be perfect and you do not need to be close to your personal fitness or health goals to embrace today as the day where you give yourself permission to be fully at home, and fully confident, in your own skin. Make the decision to pursue this true physical definition of confidence and start emulating the seven French secrets. Soon thereafter you will find yourself walking with a new mastery of vocabulary in the thoughts you think about your body and you might even need to start a new personal journal to track your monumental shift in confidence.

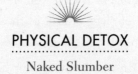

PHYSICAL DETOX
Naked Slumber

My friends in France were very open about their bodies, something foreign to my previous experience in the United States. Even the locker rooms at gyms in France were a far cry from the private experience that one expects from an American gym. The showers were communal and the changing area was open—it was impossible not to be fully exposed. The open and nonchalant acceptance of nudity opened my eyes to seeing how these women had learned to accept and embrace the skin they're in: they had never learned to be ashamed of themselves or to hide their bodies. As a result, I started intentionally doing more to let my body feel that same freedom, so, even though it was uncomfortable for me at first, I started spending more time being naked. Your physical detox portion for this chapter is to do the same.

Embrace your skin by learning to accept yourself fully—that is, without shame or judgment—in the nude. A very simple first step in doing this is to create a habit of sleeping naked. Additionally, when you wake up in the morning, allow yourself just one or two minutes to remain in your all-natural state by stretching. This simple exercise will get you more comfortable just being in the skin you're in, with nothing to hide behind. As you connect more with your birthday suit you will find yourself in a new place of natural self-acceptance.

MENTAL DETOX
Everyday Awareness

I discovered confidence because I became more in tune to understanding exactly what it was that I was looking for. In the same way, you can develop more natural confidence by increasing your day-to-day awareness and your understanding of what it is that you aspire to emulate.

A detox to help clarify your awareness skills, the following exercise will help you remove the static that causes us to be distracted in everyday life.

Reflect for a moment and think about someone you admire. Next, take a pen and use the space provided below to write out every attribute about this person that is positive and that draws you toward them. Get as specific as possible. As you write down those attributes, try to describe exactly what it is about that specific character trait that you find so attractive and alluring. After you have completed this reflection exercise, think about a second person of equal admiration in your mind and repeat the exercise.

Person One:

    Attribute One: ....

    Attribute Two: ....

    Attribute Three: ....

    Attribute Four: ....

    Attribute Five: ....

Person Two:

    Attribute One: ....

    Attribute Two: ....

    Attribute Three: ....

    Attribute Four: ....

    Attribute Five: ....

As you look at these lists, which attributes do both people share? What differentiates them? How can you emulate their example and learn from the way they live their lives and carry themselves?

SPIRITUAL DETOX
Inspiring Confidence in Others

You didn't choose me. I chose you. I appointed you to go and produce lasting fruit, so that the Father will give you whatever you ask for, using my name. (John 15:16)

Inspiring confidence in others is a by-product of the example in life that you set. The way you carry yourself—and the words you speak to others—have the power to do the same thing to others that French women did for me. When we sow words of life in those around us, we will receive them back through the reverberations of our own minds. Positivity breeds more positivity, and building confidence in others breeds more confidence in yourself. God created us to bear fruit of the spirit that would be visible and uplifting to others, and it is our obligation to share our fruit.

Below are some simple ways in which you can intentionally inspire confidence in, and share your fruit with others:

- Shower others with words of life.
- Be the first person to say something nice.
- Compliment someone on something every time you see him or her.
- Initiate meaningful conversations.
- Address and praise people for what seems obvious but is probably often overlooked.
- Express gratitude—and go out of your way to do so.

- Slow down and add more time for others in your life.
- Say hello to every person you see, and if you can, say hello by first name.
- Encourage anyone to be active by telling them how great they are doing and how great they look doing it.

....

Father, I want to honor my body with the respect and love it deserves. Forgive me for my harsh self-criticism and self-judgment and show me how to truly find freedom and beauty in the skin I'm in. I know I have only one body for life and I want to honor You with it. I am grateful for and celebrate the body You have given me. In the freeing name of Jesus, Amen.

PESSIMISTIC PERSPECTIVE

*The Truth: Life is beautiful and God
wants you to live it to the fullest.*

**Confidence allows us to love life in new ways, tasting and
savoring just how beautiful the little things about life are.**

In Love with Life

It is possible to be in love with life. In fact, that is what abundant life means and it is the type of living God wants for us. An abundance mind-set is birthed out of enthusiasm, and an enthusiastic heart is exactly what makes my best friend Melissa so in love with life. Whenever I don't quite feel like myself, I think of Melissa's attitude toward life and model my mind-set similarly. Shortly thereafter I am out of my funk and my heart is back to normal.

I started learning from Melissa when I was in college. We were on the swim team together and were close friends from day one of freshman year. Both French majors, we traveled to France for our junior year to live and study. Our parents had generously bought us each a Euro Rail pass, giving us unlimited travel access to ten different countries. We filled each weekend with adventures of hiking, exploring, and staying in hostels.

Our best trips weren't planned. We would arrive at our local train station with a backpack, a bottle of wine, and a bunch of enthusiasm. Without a destination, we jumped onto whichever train suited our fancy. We lived with freedom and let the wind blow us around. We traveled with our hearts, not our brains, and as a result, we experienced Europe in a marvelously magical way.

There were rules to how we traveled. Neither of us believed in complaining and we agreed to appreciate every detail, the highs and lows, of our adventure. Another rule was to always have the attitude of optimism no matter what happened. We traveled with unwavering enthusiasm and smiles on our faces.

On one weekend we unexpectedly ended up in Belgium. We had hopped onto the wrong train, turned ourselves around in Germany, and then landed upon the town of Bruges. The capital of the Flemish region of Belgium, Bruges is also known as the Venice of the North, as it is a canal-based city. Melissa and I rented bicycles, boated in the canal, picnicked in the cobblestoned city center, and indulged in the decadent masterpiece that is Belgian chocolate.

It was a chilly November. Bundled up in our hiking jackets, we perused the city center at night under streetlamps, people-watching as our evening entertainment. Melissa and I were poor travelers. Most of our money was depleted paying for hostels. Our evening entertainment was a city-stroll to experience as much culture as we could get for free.

On this one particular walk, life seduced us. We walked

next to the canal, across from restaurant windows glowing with silhouettes of families inside. Suddenly, a deep autumn wind came and swept up a whirlwind of leaves. As the orange, red, and burnt bark colors swirled around us, a tangible sense of peace overcame us both. We turned toward each other and laughed. "This is perfect," we agreed. Simultaneously, we both experienced an immense amount of gratitude and pure love for life. It was almost supernatural, that shared and seemingly tangible peace Melissa and I had experienced. It was a moment that couldn't be bought and can't be replicated. It had to be lived. It was a moment that can be relayed to others but never truly experienced without having been there.

I'm sure you have had a similar moment. A moment so beautiful it remains frozen in the time bank of your memory. These are often ordinary moments framed in such a way that they form picture postcards in our reflections. They open our hearts to see life differently.

There's a secret code to unlocking your heart—the way you see life—and it's already inside of you. It is your childlike enthusiasm. This type of enthusiasm is the secret to loving life. You may have repressed it, but it is still there, waiting to be awakened. You don't need a Euro Rail or an evening in Bruges to access it, because it can be aroused anywhere and doesn't depend upon location, who you are with, or the cost of an experience. It is never too late to get your childlike enthusiasm back. You just need to start playing with life again, and as you do, your enthusiasm will rekindle.

Enthusiasm is the ability to appreciate what you have, where you are, and what you are experiencing. Without enthusiasm life drags—it is a burden and a series of disconnected events. With it, life overflows with wonder, with awe, with mystery, with potential happiness at every turn.

You can move the world with enthusiasm; but before you move the world, you must first move yourself. To move yourself you must move your heart by engaging its enthusiasm. Learning how to let your enthusiasm shine is actually quite simple, so much so that I can put it into a formula for you. You can use the simple formula below as an equation with which to see the world with more enthusiasm each and every day.

ENTHUSIASM =

[Permission to enjoy] + [permission to be oneself] + [permission to be optimistic]

It is by giving yourself permission to enjoy the world around you—and all circumstances that come your way—that you can put the first piece of the enthusiasm equation together. We often live so rushed, from activity to activity, that our lives become a checklist. It's hard to enjoy life as a checklist; in fact, we miss most of life by always moving from destination to destination, checking off things that we accomplish. By giving yourself permission to enjoy life you will open a door in your heart to let yourself be you. Permission to be yourself can only come from you. It is up to you to give yourself that freedom. The more you are able to be yourself, the more you will be able to enjoy the present moment in which you live.

The final component in this enthusiasm equation is the permission to be optimistic. Optimism is a type of faith that leads to gratitude and achievement. It serves as the glue that holds the first two components of the enthusiasm equation together, for it gives the solution—enthusiasm—or anticipation for the future. Optimism carries enthusiasm from being a temporary, fleeting emotion to a sustainable, and maintainable, state of mind.

I invite you back into your childlike wonder. Play with life. Be silly. Let yourself be you. Be optimistic. Smell the roses. Laugh at the beauty of the leaves. Let the wind make you twirl with joy. Dig your toes into the sand and your fingers into the grass. Find the beauty in the small details of your day-to-day life. Awaken the childlike enthusiasm napping in your heart and look at the world with a new appreciation. Stop taking the ordinary for granted when every moment has the potential to be extraordinary.

PHYSICAL DETOX

Feeling Alive from the Inside Out

The key to Melissa's joy is her attitude of enthusiasm. She is able to emotionally engage her enthusiasm because she doesn't live life rushing from obligation to obligation. She takes time to engage her senses and doesn't hesitate to celebrate what she loves when she experiences it.

Though the idea of enthusiasm sounds like it demands a high-spirited attitude all the time, it actually requires the opposite: an ability to slow down and notice what is really around you. To help you slow down, your physical detox is to take two minutes to just breathe. Your breath can literally make you feel alive from the inside out. The way that you breathe is exceedingly important to your overall health and this portion of the detox is going to help you engage in conscious, intentional breathing. Take just two minutes to focus on breathing, a simple act we perform thousands of times a day without ever noticing. Notice how it *feels* to just breathe.

To do this breathing detox, follow the steps outlined below:

Step One:

Grab a timer—either your phone or your kitchen timer—and set it to go off in two minutes. Once you start the clock, close your eyes and focus on finding your breath. Finding your breath simply means focusing on every detail of the breathing process that you can.

Step Two:

For the purposes of this detox, you are going to increase your breathing consciousness by breathing solely through your nose. As you inhale and exhale, try to extend your exhale, making it last twice as long as your inhalations. More specifically, inhale for a slow count of three, and exhale for a slow count of seven.

Step Three:

As you experience this breathing detox, be sure to breathe from your diaphragm, or from the bottom of your rib cage, and with a rhythmic pattern. Maintain a good posture while performing your breaths whether you are sitting or lying down. As you breathe open your consciousness to your body as well as to your breathing. You can open your consciousness by thinking about sending air to specific parts of your body. Can you feel your left middle toe? Can you feel oxygen traveling to your right earlobe? Let your mind travel along your bloodstream as it races from your heart to your toes and back.

MENTAL DETOX
Learning Journal

Those who have a passion for learning have a voracious appetite for life. A love of learning keeps our hearts young. Learning is the foundation of a heart in love with life because learning never stops. Since learning never stops, the heart continues to grow with each new experience, keeping it engaged, excited, and enthusiastic. Young hearts live life with enthusiasm and passion; they live life to the fullest.

Your mental detox is to start a learning journal. Keep your journal at your bedside table and make a habit of writing down the most interesting thing you learned that day. The process of actively writing out what you learned will encourage you to look for more things to learn. The more we learn, the more actively engaged our minds will be, and, as a result, the more engrossed in life we will be. Learning is the foundation of a heart in love with life.

SPIRITUAL DETOX
Play Time

The thief's purpose is to steal and kill and destroy. My purpose is to give them a rich and satisfying life. (John 10:10)

I'm convinced that as adults we take life too seriously, and the best way to combat seriousness is with silliness. Silliness is simply an approach to opening up your inner child. It happens when we allow ourselves to be ourselves—we give ourselves permission to not care about what anyone else thinks—and we just enjoy whatever it is we are doing with a childlike openness. And yes, I seriously believe that silliness can be spiritual. In fact, God Himself is the author of joy. And we all can agree, laughter, fun, and silliness are simply expressions of joy.

Your spiritual detox is to plan something very fun for yourself and your family in the next seven days. Before your specific day of play, pray over your experience and prepare your heart to simply have a day where you enjoy being alive. You can think of this as a mini-retreat, but a retreat that isn't focused on relaxation, but rather fun. If your schedule is booked and you are unable to "get away," then play a simple game of hide-and-seek at home or flashlight tag at night. Let yourself laugh, let yourself giggle, and let yourself act like a kid again. Give praise to God for authoring laughter and fun. Here are some ideas to inspire your fun:

- Go geocaching with your family—download a

compass and geocaching app on your smartphone, pack some trail mix, and make it a day of
exploration.

- Find a lake and bring a fishing pole.
- Play a game of candle-lit Scrabble on your deck
  at night.
- Pack a picnic basket and a book and find a field
  where you can sprawl out for a few hours.
- Attend a local minor league baseball game, buy
  peanuts and Crackerjacks, and root for the
  home team.
- Set up a campfire in your backyard and spend a
  night watching the sunset and telling stories.
- Create a family field day with games like the egg
  toss, the three-legged relay, and capture the flag.
- Drive to a local city and explore it by finding.
  three museums, three monuments, and three
  locally loved cafés, restaurants, or hangouts.
- Take a Sunday afternoon drive—by yourself or
  with your family—roll the car windows down
  and blast your favorite music, drive around
  backcountry roads aimlessly and without purpose, and just enjoy being out in nature.
- If you have access to a beach, go "ghost crabbing"
  when it is pitch black at night. Take a walk on
  the beach, without flashlights or light from your
  phone, and you will see these silver dollar–sized
  transparent crabs glowing against the sand as
  they scurry to and fro.

....

Father, You promise us abundant life and I believe it is available to me. Reveal to me how to live with more joy, more confidence, more gratitude, and more abundance that my life might be a living testimony to Your love and Your glory. In the glorious name of Jesus, Amen.

A BORING LIFE

*The Truth: You have a legacy to leave
and your story matters.*

*The best way to leave a legacy that lasts is to live wholeheartedly,
making your best effort to live out the unique song of your life.*

How to Leave a Legacy

I have a friend who marches to the beat of her own drummer. Almost a decade my junior, Moe is an unlikely friend for me. I am preppy, ride a bicycle, and love the color pink. Moe has more tattoos than I can count, rides a motorcycle, and can pull off a neon green punk hairstyle. I am drawn to Moe because she is drawn to life. Life is short and precious, and Moe knows it. This attitude makes everything about Moe sparkle. She sparkles with unbridled enthusiasm, always looking for the silver lining in any cloud, and it is her sparkle that inspires others to shine in the same way.

Often considered an "old soul," Moe is an example of how age has nothing to do with our legacy. You see, she discovered the sparkle at a young age. Moe decided years ago that she wanted to live life in such a way that she could tell great stories. The legacy Moe decided to leave is one that speaks of a life well lived; she discovered that in order to live, one must live with a fully engaged heart of enthusiasm toward each and every day. Moe believes in quality. She lets her soul sing. She stops to smell the roses, she plays with puppies on the sidewalk, and she generously throws out high-fives to everyone she sees. She is committed to relishing the joys of daily life, and because of the delight she takes in life, she radiates confidence and happiness.

Moe lives with urgency, but at an even pace, enjoying life but not rushing through it. I call this mature enthusiasm. That means she is up for anything that comes her way, willing to take risks and face her fears, all without rushing or living with so much distraction that she misses out on the beautiful, small details of life. Want to fly to Las Vegas on a whim? Moe is your girl. Want to spend the afternoon rescuing turtles that are crossing the roads? Moe is your girl. Want to crash a wedding and steal the spotlight on the dance floor? Moe is your girl. Want to drive for hours in order to find the perfect picnic spot in the mountains? Moe is your girl. Want to try a new sport but are nervous about being awkward and on your own? Moe is your girl. Want to try funky foods or a new restaurant? Moe is your girl. Want to take a car ride to drive to a new state just to try out a famous ice cream shop? Moe is your girl. Want to always feel welcomed and get a high-five that is guaranteed to brighten your day? Moe is your girl.

And that is what I call engaged living. That is the type of living in which legacies are made. That is the type of living that maximizes and actually increases the longevity of your days and leaves a lasting legacy—that is a life worth telling a story about.

Moe asks herself and, by her example, asks others the following questions:

- *Is what I'm doing today going to increase the quality of my life tomorrow?*
- *How much enjoyment have I been able to squeeze out of the day today?*
- *Am I honoring my body—eating well and moving well—so that my body will last me well into my old age?*
- *Will I regret missing out on a potential great story to tell by not participating in something or by letting my fear about something hold me back?*
- *Do I live with authentic gratitude and do I express my joy thoroughly?*
- *How can I share my enthusiasm for life with others by loving them more effectively?*
- *In what ways did I really live all-out today? How did I maximize the gift that today is?*
- *Did I hold anything back?*
- *What have I loved about the journey of life today?*
- *What great stories—and what adventures—have I created with the little details of my life today that I will enjoy telling my grandchildren about?*
- *How did I invite others into the adventure of life alongside me today?*

In short, these questions paint a legacy. They are what lead to the fulfillment of "The Dash," that is, the years that represent our lives. In my case, it will be the line in between the years 1983 and 2083 (I am confidently assuming I will live to be 100 years old). This dash is a small line that encompasses my entire life, from birth to death. It is within this dash that lays my real legacy. Most tombstones typically have space for just a small phrase or a few words underneath the dash. These words are the summary of the dash; they are the words that encapsulate a lifetime of living, of impact and stories. Moe and I care about the dash that will exist on our tombstones. It is that dash that drives us both and connects our kindred spirits together as fast friends.

Live with the end in sight, for, if you do, you will live fully and without regret. Knowing your dash, or the words that will represent your dash on your tombstone, is a simple way to keep the end in sight so that you don't lose the potential of your legacy in the humdrum of the day-to-day. My tombstone, and my "dash" beneath the dash itself, will say:

TRISH BLACKWELL SYNAN

1983–2083

Wife, Mother, Daughter, Friend, Inspired Millions to Love More

While predetermining your tombstone might seem morbid, I believe it is an essential exercise in order to actually engage fully in living. It's difficult to appreciate the present unless you keep close to heart the awareness that the present will one day end. Since we are not guaranteed tomorrow, we must live the days we are given with urgency. It has been said that you never really know how to live until you first know the taste of death. Don't wait to taste death until you decide to live. You can taste death by simply acknowledging its inevitability. Death is a definite. It is part of life. It is unavoidable. Real life, on the other hand, isn't. Living—the actual act of engaging in life fully—is a choice, an active decision that depends on us. And since we know that we will die, let us also make the decision that we will really live.

Deepen your legacy by deciding right now what it is you wish to be remembered for. We are not guaranteed tomorrow, so the only way we can maximize today is to embrace today with our full selves and our full engagement. This type of full living means slowing down, increasing our daily level of gratitude, and stepping out to try new things in life. Create your own path by trusting yourself and the things that have been put on your heart.

When you live like Moe, with full engagement, enthusiasm, and a clear vision of your dash, you get the gift of living life with confidence, hope, and expectancy. In other words, you get to live with joy in how you are and how life is at that moment, and with eagerness toward what is next to come. Tattoo your life with permanency by living a life worth telling a story about.

PHYSICAL DETOX
Maximized Alkalinity

An often-overlooked element of optimal physical health is the natural internal pH balance of our gastrointestinal system. Everything that we eat or drink has either an acidic or alkaline impact on our digestive system. Ideally, our gastrointestinal system operates at its highest efficiency when neutrally balanced, meaning that it has an equal amount of acidic and alkaline inputs that offset one another to create a neutral environment. Unfortunately, a large amount of our modern diet is based around foods that are acidifying once ingested. When our internal pH is out of balance, particularly with an acidic imbalance, we incur negative physical side effects. In particular, the negative effects of an acidic imbalance in our bodies can result in inflammation in the body, disruption of the digestive track, insomnia, frequent headaches, water retention, low blood pressure, fatigue, gastritis, leg cramps, frequent infections, and depression. In addition to the gastrointestinal benefit of an optimal pH balance, an increase in alkaline input can be beneficial in helping to decrease one's propensity to osteoporosis.

It is important to be intentional about incorporating more alkaline-producing foods into our diet to help prevent internal pH acidity. The best foods for alkaline production are dark, leafy vegetables, lemon or lime juice, and fruit with a low glycemic index such as apples, grapefruits, bananas, and oranges. Avoid or minimize consumption of high-acidifying foods such as meat, fish, eggs, grains, legumes, peppermint, chocolate, and alcohol.

This week pick three dark, leafy vegetables or alkalinizing vegetables to add to your diet. Buy enough of all three to be able to have some of each with your dinner each night of the week. Some options to choose from are broccoli, dandelions, mushrooms, onions, peppers, pumpkin, radishes, rutabaga, spinach, green beans, eggplant, cucumber, wheat grass, sweet potatoes, tomatoes, and kale.

MENTAL DETOX
Your Dash

It's your turn to write your life out backward.

Your dash should be twelve words or less and it should encapsulate everything that means the most to you in your life. This mental exercise seems simple in concept, but it is very emotionally challenging to do and difficult to execute. Do not be discouraged if you struggle to find the perfect way to phrase your dash; just write a dash to start and know that you can always rewrite and improve the wording of your dash at a later date. Your dash should include something about who you are and something about the impact and legacy you are leaving.

As you consider your dash, ask yourself the following questions:

- *What is it that I want to be remembered for?*
- *Who do I want to be remembered by?*
- *How long do I hope to live?*
- *What will my great-great-grandchildren be able to say about me?*
- *How can I summarize the legacy I hope for in the most succinct phrase possible?*
- *How far-reaching will my influence be, and how many lives will be touched by mine?*
- *What values matter the most to me and how will my legacy reflect those?*
- *What are the exact words my tombstone will say?*

Write out your dash in the space below. Then memorize it and write it on your heart. Additionally, take a piece of paper and write your dash on it, posting it where you will see it every day. The more you can do to keep your dash at the forefront of your mind, the more clarity and encouragement you will have as you live your day-to-day life.

_____

(Your Name)

_____ - _____

(Your birth year and death year)

_____

(The phrase that summarizes your dash)

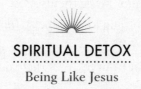

SPIRITUAL DETOX

Being Like Jesus

Imitate God, therefore, in everything you do, because you are his dear children. Live a life filled with love, following the example of Christ. He loved us and offered himself as a sacrifice for us, a pleasing aroma to God. (Ephesians 5:1–2)

We are given the gift of being able to watch and then emulate other people's lives and examples. Watching Moe live life well has helped me learn how to live life well.

The ultimate example of the person Who lived life to the fullest was Jesus. Jesus loved people. He went to parties, hung out with the rejected, and broke the rules of society when necessary. His legacy is the greatest legacy of all. He is the person we should all aspire to emulate and become like.

The greatest commandment Jesus ever gave is to love and to love with all our hearts. In John 13:34 He said, "So now I am giving you a new commandment: Love each other. Just as I have loved you, you should love each other." The best way we can become like Jesus is to love another more. Be like Jesus by being intentional and generous with your love this week. Over the next twenty-four hours make it your intention to love radically. Radical love is displayed through small acts of meaningful love; below are some suggestions to help you get started on your twenty-four-hour love fest:

- Write a thank-you note to someone you love to thank them for being themselves.
- Donate something to your local Goodwill or Red Cross.
- Forgive a hurt from the past that you have held on to.
- Bake banana bread for all the neighbors on your street and put it in their mailbox with a bow on it.
- Volunteer your time to a homeless shelter or food kitchen.
- Put away someone else's grocery cart for them in the parking lot.
- Hold the door for a mom with her hands full.
- Buy coffee for the person behind you in line.
- Send a $50 bill in the mail to a stranger with no return address on the envelope.

- Offer to mow your neighbor's lawn for them when you mow yours.
- Ask your cashier how their day really is going and listen well to what they say.
- Call up an old friend you haven't spoken to in a while just to say hello.
- Compliment everyone you see on something beautiful about them.
- Be a word of encouragement to your partner, thanking them for all they do for you.
- Do a chore around the house that typically is your partner's responsibility.
- Offer to babysit for a couple so they can have a date night out together.
- Buy five copies of your favorite and most encouraging book and send it to five friends.

....

Father, thank You for teaching me that I matter, and because I matter, my story matters. Let me not take for granted that how I live my life tells a story, and leave a legacy. I pray for wisdom and love that I might be a true imitator of Christ and leave a mark on this world that encourages others to do the same. In the beloved name of Jesus, Amen.

NARROW WORLDVIEW

The Truth: Confidence is available to you.

Little changes in our internal vocabulary cause big changes to occur.

A Sheepish Shift in Perspective

In Greece, we drove an airport rental, a little Fiat Panda. Typical of a small European car, the Fiat barely had the engine power to get up the rolling hills of the Greek countryside that spread before us. Puttering along the cliffside road from the southernmost tip of the Attica peninsula, we traveled from Sounion, the site of the majestic Temple of Poseidon, back to the city of Athens being chased by the setting sun. Nick navigated Brandon and me through the single-lane roads of the local villages to avoid potential city traffic on the main highway. Enveloped by the twilight shadows of dusk we soaked up the last remnants of sunlight after a day filled with sightseeing, wine tasting, and fresh seafood.

Without warning, Nick slammed the breaks on the Fiat.

The sunlight had tricked his vision and we found ourselves in a rural traffic jam.

We were surrounded by sheep—hundreds of them. Somehow our Fiat positioned itself at the center of their flock as the herd crossed the small dirt road. Our little blue Panda was but a polka dot in a spread of white wool. I pressed my face up to the car window and laughed at the absurdity of it all. We were stuck. No movement forward. No movement backward. There were sheep everywhere.

That evening over glasses of Nimean wines the three of us couldn't stop giggling about our run-in with the sheep. It was Brandon's first time abroad, and as he recalls the experience he explains the sheep engulfment as *the* moment his frame of reference about the world expanded.

Our frames of reference are the vision through which we see the world and what is possible within that world. The frame we set up for ourselves determines the boundaries of our minds, our imaginations, and our potential. So, as our frame of what is possible expands, so, too, does what is actually possible expand as well. The expansion of our vision doesn't demand radical changes in our thoughts, but instead, a simple shift of adjustment, as in a slight zoom out of a camera lens.

It's impossible to see an entire picture if you are zoomed in; to see the full potential of what is before you, you must be zoomed out. In the same way, to see and chase our full personal potential, we need our frames to be zoomed out in such a way that we can see the possibility of what lies before us. Many people never reach their full potential in life because they expect perfection out of themselves—they are too zoomed in and have been convinced that the fulfillment of their potential is entirely up to them. As this is an unrealistic expectation, they inevitably fail or fall short and experience discouragement. They want change in their lives, but the change is often so drastic that it's intimidating or impossible to maintain. Subsequently, the moment the change becomes too difficult, discouragement sets in and growth stops.

Real change doesn't happen overnight. It isn't radical but rather happens in small shifts and tiny adjustments. Weight loss is a slow, progressive process. Shaping your thoughts to become more positive is a daily endeavor in mental training. Pursuing a lifelong dream takes years of small, bold decisions and actions. Financial security for retirement is achieved over many years of making wise decisions with money, debt, and investments. Anything worth pursuing in life takes time and likewise we must be patient as we pursue our potential and purpose.

What happened on that rural Greek road at sunset wasn't radical, but it changed how Brandon saw the world in a radical way. Those sheep opened his eyes to a new comprehension of cultures, of what is possible and what exists outside his normal American day-to-day life. They taught him that there was so much more to the world than he had previously ever imagined. The clash of modernity with ancient tradition challenged what he thought he knew about the world outside of his Washington, D.C., suburb. As so often is the case, it's not the big things that change us, but the small things.

Changes in our thought lives and mind-sets don't occur as a result of radical changes in our lives either, but rather they happen as a result of small and deliberate shifts in our thinking. In the same way, our understanding of ourselves and of God's great plan for us can be expanded by similar small adjustments.

The journey to understand the gifts, talents, and passions given to us by God builds our confidence about who we were created to be. Confidence is yours, available to you with a simple expansion of your perspective. There is no radical change that needs to happen, rather a day-by-day transformation of seeing ourselves as God sees us. It is through small changes that we improve, and likewise, a small shift in perspective can be the catalyst for personal growth. The vocabulary of our minds is reconstructed through the daily discipline of paying attention to the words we speak to ourselves. By not allowing limited thinking, or a small-framed mind-set, we open our vocabulary to become more expansive. The more expansive our internal vocabulary, the more we can live freely with the limitlessness that God gives us.

You can shift your frame of reference in how you see the world through meditating on and refining your belief about God and about what He has planned for you. Deepen your faith and confidence by strengthening the framework of your mind-set with:

- Belief that God will complete the good work (potential) He started in you (Philippians 1:6).
- Belief in God's abundance (2 Corinthians 9:8).
- Belief that God is good (Psalm 136:1).
- Belief that God is for you and not against you (Romans 8:31).
- Belief that God can expand our frame of the world (Ephesians 3:17–19).
- Belief that we are a work-in-progress under God's close supervision (Philippians 1:6).

- Belief that there is beauty in the world every-where we look (Psalm 19:1).
- Belief that your past does not define you but instead refines you (2 Corinthians 5:17).
- Belief that your story matters (Psalm 107:2).
- Belief that you are being transformed more and more every day (Romans 12:2).
- Belief that God has a plan for you (Jeremiah 29:11).

Your potential exceeds your imagination. Embrace the good news that you don't need to make radical changes to direct yourself toward that potential, but instead, it is in small ways that you are transformed day by day. Each day is an opportunity to become a better version of yourself, and by focusing on just that you will be delighted by moments of life when sheep engulf your world and your frame gets expanded.

PHYSICAL DETOX
Fiber Up!

One way to see a small positive change in your physical health is by ensuring that you get the recommended daily allotment (RDA) of fiber in your diet. According to the USDA, the RDA for fiber intake is 25 grams per day for women and 38 grams per day for men. In contrast, most adults actually eat only an average of 15 grams of fiber per day. Lack of dietary fiber leads not only to constipation, but also to a decrease in the efficiency of the digestive system. The long-term effect of a compromised digestive system can be devastating and includes potential issues such as a heightened propensity for gastrointestinal issues, heart disease, diabetes, and stroke.

Make fiber a priority in your diet this week. As you do your regular weekly grocery shopping, add to your shopping cart five additional foods that are high in fiber (and that you don't normally buy). Add one extra serving of fiber from these foods each day of the coming week and you will begin to start climbing your way to the recommended daily allotment of fiber.

To help you decide which five foods to add to your shopping list this week, here are a few fiber champions: beans, peas, whole wheat flour, raspberries, blackberries, prunes, dark leafy vegetables, sweet potatoes, carrots, pumpkin, cabbage, oats, bananas, blueberries, broccoli, kale, spinach, cauliflower, snap peas, asparagus, corn, cornmeal, wheat germ, wheat bran, lentils, and fibrous fruits.

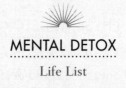

MENTAL DETOX
Life List

As your frame of the world starts to expand, so, too, will your personal frame for your potential grow. The possibility of what is ahead of you is limitless if you believe that God can use your life and your story to show off His glory.

Dream big today and create your "Five for Life" list. This is a list of the five biggest dreams that are on your heart. They are five things that you would want to do or accomplish if you had absolutely nothing holding you back. These are things that you would pursue wholeheartedly if you knew confidently that you could not fail. Think big and use the space below to create your list:

1) ....
2) ....
3) ....
4) ....
5) ....

Writing these dreams down should feel scary and exhilarating at the same time. For something to classify as worthy of your "Five for Life" it needs to scare you. These are dreams for which you don't have the answers or a clear understanding of the pathway toward yet—they are the seeds of dreams that have been sown in your heart. By writing them down and proclaiming them as a possibility for your life, you are claiming them within your frame of potential. You don't need to know how you will accomplish these dreams; you just need to know that you have them. All big dreams start with small seeds, and your list for this mental detox is your small seed. The great things you accomplish in life won't happen overnight, but instead will be birthed out of ideas and decisions that start with just a thought.

Now that you have the seed of your list, water your dreams by posting your "Five for Life" somewhere visible so you can see it on a daily basis. By reviewing your dreams on a daily basis you keep the dream alive and close within the framework of your vision.

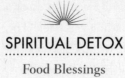

SPIRITUAL DETOX
Food Blessings

There you and your families will feast in the presence of the Lord your God, and you will rejoice in all you have accomplished because the Lord your God has blessed you. (Deuteronomy 12:7)

Saying a prayer of thanks and gratitude over a meal is a way to humbly remember that God is our provider. It is in this way that the blessing is a daily reminder to keep the framework of our gratitude expanded toward the goodness and provision of God.

If you don't do so already, start praying over your meals. Your prayers don't need to be extensive or fancy, they just need to come from a place of gratitude and praise. Once you are in the habit of praying over every dinner you eat, start praying over your lunches, and then your breakfasts. You can use the following prayer as a simple template to help you get started:

Father, I praise You for showing me that I can have confidence and that You have great things in store for me. Thank You for stretching and expanding my perspective and for reminding me that I am being renewed through the transformation of my thoughts more and more each and every day. I am so glad that You have my life in Your hands and that You will hold my hand as I walk towards fulfilling my potential and my purpose in this life. In the safe name of Jesus, Amen.

....

*Father, thank You for the food You have set out before
me and for the hands that prepared it, making it
possible for me to have this meal. Bless this food to
the nourishment of my body; may it energize me that
I might live out a life that overflows of Your love and
goodness. In the generous name of Jesus, Amen.*

LACK OF FOCUS

The Truth: God's love is the foundation of your confidence.

The right focus will frame your perspective positively so you can be confident and happy on a daily basis; living with this type of intentional thinking is the framework of confidence.

The Framework of Confidence

My wedding day in Bora Bora was perfect, the dream day I never knew I had. When I think of the most perfect day of my life, I think of that day. The day of my wedding, we woke up in our overwater bungalow and went for a run together along the island coast, soaking up the forty-four shades of blue Polynesian waters. For breakfast we sat like kings on palm thrones and were served champagne and fresh fruit with a view of Mount Otemanu. We donned white swimwear and explored the aquatic wildlife with snorkels, and then sunbathed for two hours before the hairstylist arrived to prepare me for the ceremony, which was held in an overwater chapel at sunset. Our wedding photos are so beautiful they look faked, but they are real. We retired to our castle on the water after the ceremony, before our celebration dinner. Our bungalow glowed. It was as if the Pacific waters and the twinkling stars were aligned in their reflections. The evening ended with us once again seated on palm thrones, this time beachside, for a romantic dinner of lobster and fresh-caught fish, serenaded by our own private musician.

After Brandon and I got home, I had the task of framing our bamboo papyrus marriage certificate. It is my most cherished piece of paper. Water-stained and tattered from the twenty-seven hours on boats, planes, and cars that it took to get from Bora Bora back to Virginia, the pressure to choose the right frame was intense. I wanted the memory of my wedding day to be perfectly captured, carefully protected, and beautifully displayed for the world to see. In short, I wanted that fragile piece of papyrus to be framed in a way that it would last and tell well its story. Framing it for prominent display represents my confidence in the love, promise, and potential of my marriage.

Choosing a frame for a painting, photo, or certificate can be overwhelming. The craft stores that house these frames are daunting, often with five aisles of wall-to-wall options and two additional aisles of matting selections. Add to that the corner of the store dedicated to custom framing, equipped with a staff who can transpose images of what your future framed item will look like, and estimates on the hundreds of dollars it will cost you to do so, and the options are overwhelming.

I avoid the framing process unless the item is really important to me. Whenever I venture into a craft store with a framing project in mind, I'm as prepared as one can be for these hundreds of options, which means I'm not prepared at all. The process takes hours and I am never really sure if the framing options I chose are the best, as every variation and option gives the project a completely different look.

I finally settled on a black distressed bamboo frame. The paper isn't perfect and has no real value, but what it represents is and does. That frame holds my perfect day on my wall.

In the same way my worn marriage certificate has flaws, so do we. Thankfully, God sees the tattered pieces of our lives and personalities in the same way I see my marriage certificate: as beautiful and perfect. The frame through which God sees us makes our broken pieces whole; He makes our wear-and-tear fresh and beautiful. Putting ourselves in the right frame can make all the difference in how the world sees us and in how we see the world.

The frame around us—that is, God's love—can make us (tattered pieces of paper and all) really whole. It is God's presence itself that structures love, hope, and perfection around us, almost as if the sides of the frame are His arms surrounding us in support. It is with this perspective that we can frame the way we see ourselves with confidence.

I have confidence in my frame because I have framed myself with God's strength and lined myself with the matting of His love. Confidence is a mental muscle, and, like any muscle of the body, must be worked out consistently for it to grow and strengthen. We train this confidence muscle by consciously choosing to accept ourselves as who we are—flaws, tears, imperfections, and all, because we know that the frame that surrounds us, God's frame of love and acceptance, is what makes us completely whole. When we are framed in

God's strength and love, we can overlook our weaknesses and instead be confident in the wholeness and perfect vision He allows us to have in His frame.

Whether you realize it or not, you frame your confidence in one way or another. The frame is the perspective with which you see the world, how you interpret your experiences, and the confidence you feel about your future, your potential, your worth, and your identity. Most of us live with whatever frame comes naturally to us, and usually that is a frame riddled with negativity and limitations. The good news is that good framing is available to everyone. You may need to reframe what is currently there, but thankfully the cost is reasonable and doable—the cost is our focus. The confidence frame that is offered to us by God is available to us, for free, if we simply direct our minds and our thoughts to seeing ourselves the way He sees us. True confidence comes from focusing on God and on His opinion of us. He loves us completely, accepts us fully, and has great plans for us. In the framework of His opinion, there is absolutely nothing about which we cannot feel confident.

Frame the perspective with which you see the world with optimism. One of the key components of confidence is the ability to see the silver lining of any situation. It is an ability to look at a picture and, instead of seeing the wear and damage, see the perfection and promise it represents. When we live in God's framework we get to see ourselves with that silver-lining perspective. This perspective gives us grace for our past and hope for our future in the same way that my wedding certificate encapsulates perfection and promise of love in the future through a tattered memento.

Re-frame the way you see yourself by selecting first a new frame and then a matting to compliment the frame. The frame that will best compliment you is the frame structure provided to us by God. He gives us structure and support. Framing your confidence well doesn't have to be as daunting a task as framing something in the craft store, because we have already been given the framework of confidence in our identity as children of God. Galatians 3:26 tells us we are children of God in faith, and like any child who makes art for their parent, God is proud of us. Our lives are our art, and He is our Father, eager to frame what we hand to Him for full display. Let your confidence be grounded in knowing that God loves you and is proud of you simply because you are His child. Everything you offer to Him is worthy of being framed. Frame your life with His love and every day will be filled with confidence, making it a masterpiece.

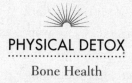

PHYSICAL DETOX
Bone Health

The literal framework of our physical bodies are our bones. Bone health is incredibly important to healthy aging and to our ability to keep our tattered selves looking beautiful. We can invest in our bone health by investing in the density of our bones. There are two major ways to contribute to your bone health: calcium supplements and strength training. Strength training in particular is essential to increasing bone density and in the prevention of osteoporosis. The good news is that no matter your current age or your experience with working out, you can strength-train and reap excellent benefits for your bones.

For optimal bone-strengthening results, make it your goal to strength-train at least three times per week for a minimum of thirty minutes per training session. You don't need access to weights or to a gym to engage in resistance training, as there are ample exercises you can do at home using your own body weight as resistance. Your physical detox for your bone health is to create a plan of action to incorporate strength training into your weekly workout schedule.

MENTAL DETOX
Time Machine Clarity

Insecurity can manifest itself as self-doubt, making it difficult for us to focus and live life with clarity. Step into a time machine to the past with me. Close your eyes after you read this paragraph and journey back into the caverns of your memory. As you reflect I want you to remember the *first* time you felt not good enough (or "not .... enough," you can fill in the blank)—your first experience of insecurity, so to speak.

Get into that moment. Close your eyes again and give yourself permission to feel. Be with that experience for a solid two minutes, keeping your eyes closed and your breath calm and smooth. The purpose of this exercise is to help you let go of your past so that you can harness a clearer focus and purpose for your future.

After you open your eyes, take just a moment to really define the details of that experience. Here are a few questions to ponder as you reflect:

> *How old were you?*
> *What were the circumstances of the situation?*
> *How did you feel before and then after you first experienced the "not _____ enough" ache?*
> *What was said to you by others?*
> *What did you say to yourself at that moment?*
> *What did you learn about yourself?*
> *How long did that experience stick with you?*
> *What do you still say to yourself about this memory?*

Below is some space for your answers. Make sure you take a few minutes to consider how letting go of some of these past hurts will free up mental and emotional space so you can move confidently toward your future.

....

....

....

....

....

SPIRITUAL DETOX
....
Soul Satisfied

For he satisfies the thirsty and fills the hungry with good things. (Psalm 107:9)

Living in the frame of God's love is the only way we will ever live with satisfied souls. Hang the artwork of your life on God's wall by offering your life to Him. On God's wall our lives always become masterpieces.

We can all learn to live with a more satisfied soul. Invest in the satisfaction of your soul by getting to know God better. As you learn more about God, you will trust the framework He provides for your life with more faith and confidence. The best way to increase your knowledge of God and ultimately satisfy your soul is by reading the words of life that God has left for us. These words are found in the Bible. The more you read the Bible and simply spend time in it, the more God will reveal your life's meaning. As your knowledge, wisdom, and meaning in life increase, your soul will find peace and satisfaction like it has never known before.

Reading the Bible is different from any other type of reading. When reading the Bible, it doesn't matter how much you read, how many chapters or verses you get through, or how long you spend reading, it just matters that you open the book and read and spend time learning from God and learning to hear Him speak to you. When you come across a verse or a phrase that catches your attention, slow down and meditate on it and its meaning.

Satisfy your soul by keeping your Bible out on your kitchen counter this week, placing it next to your coffee-maker. While your coffee brews in the morning, use that time to read God's Word.

....

Father, You are my foundation. Let everything I am and everything I do be based in You. Thank You for satisfying my soul, for quenching my thirst and for filling me and my life with Your goodness. May I never base my confidence in anything or anyone other than You. In the foundational name of Jesus, Amen.

PAST HURTS

*The Truth: The waves of your life have
created great beauty in your story.*

*The storms of our past wear into us lessons of an unbreakable
nature that transform us into beautiful treasures.*

Weathering Waves
···

As a kid I walked the sands of the Jersey Shore with intensity,
looking through patches of washed-up seashells. It wasn't the
seashells I was after though, I was in pursuit of something
much greater and more valuable to me: sea glass. Poking
out from behind the beige grains of sand and hidden behind
clunky shells laid a kaleidoscope of colored glass fragments.
The discovery of a piece of well-worn sea glass was a true treasure. Physically and chemically weathered by the salt water of
the ocean, the sea glass menagerie I collected was beautiful.
I shared the boasts of my treasures with my grandfather, who
also collected sea glass. We spent our afternoons speculat-
ing over the origin, the journey, and the story of that glass.
Our pieces were frosted varieties of cream, green, and blue

with fully rounded edges and smooth surfaces. What were originally broken shards of glass, these small pieces had been rolled and tumbled around in the ocean for decades—thirty years on average—before being washed up on shore for us to find. These sea glass treasures sang to me of the interconnectedness of people between decades and of the potential for something sharp and edgy to become smooth, comforting, and beautiful.

Sea glass has other names, names that far better convey the beauty I am describing: sea gems, beach jewels, mermaid tears, and sea pearls, among others. These are certainly powerful names for something that was once discarded trash.

In the same way that the ocean recycles our trash—our broken pieces of glass—so, too, is the trash of our lives used and recycled by God to create something of beauty. We have all been sharp and edgy, and like sea glass, we all have the potential for these rough edges to be smoothed out by the waves of life. These waves batter us around, but beyond the roughness and the rocking is a final outcome, a product of beauty, that could not have ever existed without the waves.

Like real sea glass I have been tousled around in the throes of thirty years of life. It has taken some very rough storms to soften and shape my edges, and even more squalls for me to realize the beauty that was forming in me as a result of the pain, hurt, disappointment, failure, rejection, fear, suffering, and uncertainty I experienced. Over time I finally started to see the beauty that was being shaped within me, and as a result, my story started to have a different kind of shine to it.

The waves of our lives are exactly what are responsible for

the beauty we carry. Without the waves we would be sharp, discarded glass pieces, but the waves transform us. And while they aren't always gentle, they always leave us strong. A regular piece of glass shatters when it is dropped on the floor, but a piece of sea glass is fortified and thickened—it is not easily broken.

What are the waves in your story that have made you feel tossed around? What waves have rocked your life? In thinking about my waves, and my story, I used to think some waves and storms trashed my life, like a giant hurricane that left me disheveled and broken. I was rocked by financial uncertainty, unhappiness between my parents, emotional rejection, an anxiety disorder, insecurity, self-destructive habits, sexual assault and ensuing post-traumatic stress disorder—and the waves rolled on. They battered me, they beat me, but they did not defeat me.

I now see the waves differently. I now see the purpose in their undercurrent. I now see how they have weathered my spirit to a place of beauty and confidence, as they sanded into me lessons I would have not otherwise ever had the opportunity to learn.

Your waves are something in which you can be confident. They have left you frosted, smooth, and unbreakable. Your waves have made your story worth telling.

Be confident in the weathered version of you. The waves have molded you, smoothed over your sharp edges, and brought you to new shores of life that you may have never considered possible before. My sea glass collection hails from all over the world, but each piece landed on the sands of the Jersey Shore. When you ride the waves of life with confidence in the beauty that is being etched by the sand, you, too, will arrive at new lands you never expected.

Furthermore, the waves boast of your strength and resilience, they are in fact all the proof you need that you have something to be confident about: your safety in God's arms. Our life waves carry us deeper into confidence by deepening our confidence in the God Who carries us through the storms.

The best part about this frosted beauty we each carry is that we aren't responsible for it. We don't need to know where the waves are taking us or what will come out of our next round of smoothing; we just need to know that God knows. He directs the waves. He blows on the ocean. He steers our brokenness to shores of beauty and takes what is broken to make it beautiful beyond measure. He turns our gashes into gems, our junk into jewels, and our tears into pearls.

Rejoice with me that with every year that passes we will become only more weathered—and thereby beautiful and fortified—and that is something to feel confident about.

PHYSICAL DETOX
Aged Beauty

The mark of true beauty is the ability to embrace and celebrate one's body, not just at any age, but at every age. Though it may not seem like it superficially, the body does become more beautiful with age. Its beauty comes from the stories it is able to tell. The wrinkling and weathering that happens over time enriches the natural beauty that therein lies.

Some questions for reflection as you consider the beauty of your body and as you prepare your mind to start seeing older bodies for the extra beauty they carry:

- What do you know now about your body that you didn't know twenty years ago?
- Where has your body carried you?
- How has your body been faithful and trusty through the waves of life?
- What scars does your body boasts that speak stories about your life?
- Your body tells a story, what does yours say?
- Can you think of someone who is older than you whose body is absolutely beautiful in its wrinkled and weathered state?

Your ability to become more beautiful physically over time is dependent upon your attitude toward aging and on the words you speak to yourself about your aging body. If you can celebrate your body for how it has carried you and for the experiences it has endured, then you will start to see the aged beauty that has been carefully crafted. Write your body a love letter from the perspective of you being well into old age. Thank your body for what it has done for you, take note of its resilience, and celebrate it for the story it has told as it has carried you successfully through life:

Dear Beautiful Body,

....

....

....

....

....

Love,

....

MENTAL DETOX

The Million-Dollar Challenge

One of the best things about the waves of our lives is that they equip us to love and empathize with others with more sincerity. As you consider the waves that have hit you the most harshly in your life, think about how they make you passionate about wanting to help others. My personal storm of lacking confidence and battling an eating disorder have made me passionate about helping women and men feel alive, free, and amazing in the skin they're in. Additionally my heart is softened toward helping women who have been victims of sexual crimes and oppression after I myself experienced sexual assault. I am convinced that our waves open our hearts to feel compassion in ways toward others that we never could have known otherwise. Through these seemingly devastating waves we learn how to express love to others in a way that is possible only because we had walked through a similar type of pain ourselves.

If you were to receive one million dollars today with the stipulation that you couldn't keep the money, but had to give it all away, to whom would you give it? Looking at the full story of our lives and our waves gives us perspective on the types of outreach and people we most want to help.

To whom would you give away a million dollars, and why?

Come up with an answer to this question today and then, within a week of reading this, do something to contribute to that cause. It doesn't have to be big, just do something.

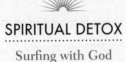

SPIRITUAL DETOX
Surfing with God

But You, O Lord, are a God of compassion and mercy, slow to get angry and filled with unfailing love and faithfulness. (Psalm 86:15)

My brother-in-law John Brian, a Young Life leader involved in high school ministry and mentorship, lives at the beach because he was placed there on assignment, but also because he loves to surf. John Brian doesn't surf alone; he surfs with his man Jesus. He goes out at the break of day and spends time on his board in prayer, reflection, and fellowship with God. And John Brian knows something about waves—he has been through many in his life that have rocked him hard, and yet, just like in his experience of actual surfing, he has found that Jesus has carried him, not just through, but on top of the waves.

What waves in your life has God carried you through?

When you look back at your waves, can you see yourself surfing with God? Instead of looking at the waves that come as storms, imagine yourself as a thrill-seeking surfer who gets to ride giant waves with Jesus.

Take a moment and reflect on the most recent wave that has rocked your life. As you think back on the circumstances and challenges of that wave, as well as the growth you experienced in the outcome, envision yourself surfing on top of the wave instead of being thrown around by the wave.

....

Father, how beautiful are the waves of the storms in my life that have shaped my sharp edges and pains into something soft and beautiful. I praise You for taking what would normally be discarded and creating out of it something of value. Thank You for letting nothing in my life be wasted and thank You for showing me the beauty You can craft out of my past pains. In the artful name of Jesus, Amen.

LACK OF ROUTINE

The Truth: Confidence is something you renew daily.

**To maximize the effectiveness of this book, go back over the detox
exercises on a daily basis. Make them a part of your lifestyle.**

Conquering Life with Confidence

I said this earlier, but I am obsessed with having a clean mouth.
And while I do care about the language that comes out of my
mouth, I'm not talking about that kind of clean mouth. I love
having clean teeth and minty-fresh breath. As a result, I pride
myself on my dental hygiene. I brush and use mouthwash
three times daily. I have perfectly straight and white teeth,
without ever having had braces. I've always known my smile is
one of my best assets, so I tend to my teeth accordingly. I take
pride in my teeth.

And, as they say, pride comes before a fall.

You can imagine my surprise, and my shame, when the
dentist recently told me I had eight cavities. I thought it was a
joke. It wasn't.

As it turns out, I'm not a good flosser. Perhaps I should re-phrase that: I'm good at flossing; I just did it "frequently," not daily. I'm a frequent flosser, and I thought that counted for something; just like frequent flyers get extra perks, I assumed I did, too. The sad truth is that I knew this was coming. My bedtime ritual with my husband was always a little off. We would start brushing our teeth together and I would be in bed, teeth cared for, face washed, and pajamas put on before he even finished flossing his teeth. He is a flossing champion. Never misses. He always told me to slow down my bedtime routine, but I was a woman on a mission: sleep. I need nine hours a night and Brandon only needs six to seven, so I took getting to bed before him seriously. That is, until the dentist gave me the cavity news.

When he confirmed it wasn't a joke, I asked how it could have happened. And then the question came:

Are you flossing daily?

Yikes. Daily? How about frequently? We both knew the answer.

Those extra hours I spent having my cavities filled gave me a lot of time to think about the difference between doing something frequently versus doing it daily. When it comes to things that need maintenance and cleaning, like our teeth and our minds, frequent attention does not suffice. In our mouths, the buildup of plaque can lead to tooth decay and gum dis-ease. Flossing, brushing, and using mouthwash—all three of those things—daily will help prevent the destructive buildup of plaque. In the same way, we need to floss, brush, and wash out our minds. Plaque is the harmful buildup of germs that live in the mouth and on teeth. Mental plaque is the harmful buildup of fear, insecurity, self-doubt, negativity, and anxiety that live in the brain and on our thoughts.

When we floss our mental facilities we are looking to get in between the thoughts that we've had, in between the circumstances we experience, and in between the lines of our stories in order to extract the real meaning of our day. After we have flossed for meaning, we scrub our minds with brushes that wash away any negativity, self-doubt, or fear clinging to our brain. And finally, we wash our minds clear by swishing around fresh new ideas and positive affirmations that we then spit out and put into action.

In the same way we need to floss our teeth daily to control plaque buildup in our mouths, we must also floss our minds daily to prevent debilitating mental plaque. Frequent application of the exercises in this book will be good for you, but they won't do the job entirely in the same way frequent flossing didn't prevent me from getting cavities. You might get a little of the decay off your mental teeth, but ultimately, without frequency, enough will stay caked on and deteriorate the pristine confidence you are meant to have.

To maximize the effectiveness of this book, go back over the detox exercises on a daily basis. Make them a part of your lifestyle. The vocabulary of your mind has changed and been super-cleaned. You've just had a full deep cleaning and now it's up to you to maintain it.

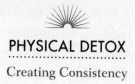

PHYSICAL DETOX
Creating Consistency

As our journey together comes to a close, it is important that I leave you with a map to success. This map is your plan to be consistent with your fitness and nutrition so that you feel confident. The more consistently we stay committed to something, the more confident we will feel about ourselves in that area. Your final physical detox is to set a schedule for your physical health and fitness. As you consider your ideal health goals, consider the following questions:

- *How many days per week are you able to commit to clean, nutritious eating?*
- *What day of the week will you do your grocery shopping so that you are always prepared with healthy options in your house?*
- *How many days per week will you commit to your workouts?*
- *What kind of cardio workouts will you do and how many times per week can you commit to doing cardio workouts?*
- *Strength and resistance training is critical for long-term bone health as well as metabolic health. How many days per week can you commit to strength training?*

By making the decision now, you are committing to yourself and increasing the probability of follow-through. Complete your final physical detox of this experience by answering the questions above thoughtfully. For optimal results, be specific about which days of the week you are able to commit to consistent workouts.

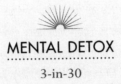

MENTAL DETOX
3-in-30

As you move forward with your new vocabulary and *Insecurity Detox*, one way to stay on top of your self-development and to keep your confidence in check is by creating three major goals and focuses for each month. By keeping it to three simple goals, you won't feel overwhelmed or distracted. Additionally, as you complete each month's goals and make progress, you will feel encouraged and empowered, giving you momentum to successfully conquer the next month's goals as well.

Take a moment to put the book down and make your first 3-in-30 right now. You can decide your three goals for the month by considering what are your most pressing or challenging things.

Make a note in your calendar or set an alarm on your phone to revisit your 3-in-30 on the last day of the month and then to create next month's 3-in-30 on the first of every month.

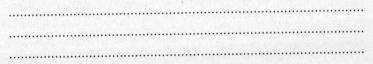

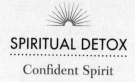

SPIRITUAL DETOX
Confident Spirit

That is why we never give up. Though our bodies are dying, our spirits are being renewed every day. For our present troubles are small and won't last very long. Yet they produce for us a glory that vastly outweighs them and will last forever! So we don't look at the troubles we can see now; rather, we fix our gaze on things that cannot be seen. For the things we see now will soon be gone, but the things we cannot see will last forever. (2 Corinthians 4:16–18)

As you complete the journey of this insecurity detox, your final spiritual detox is intended to equip you with a way to renew your confident spirit daily. The most consistent way we can conquer life with confidence is by arming ourselves with the truth about which we can be most confident: the way God loves us and works in our lives. Consider the words of Philippians 1:6:

> *And I am certain that God, who began the good work within you, will continue his work until it is finally finished on the day when Christ Jesus returns.*

These words are our assurance that God will not leave us. He will continue to walk alongside us as we progress closer and closer to becoming like Him, and He will grow us—our talents, our potential, our love, and our story—until our story is complete and our good work leaves the legacy He has intended for us.

Take the following prayer and say it at the beginning of

each day. Write it down on a piece of paper and put it on your bathroom sink next to your toothbrush until you have it memorized, and make it a habit to say this prayer at the start of every day so that you might start each day with confidence.

....

Father, thank You for creating me with potential and purpose; I confidently praise You for carrying out to completion the good work You have started in me. Deepen my love for others, overflow my heart with wisdom, and create within me a confident light of hope that the life I lead might make a difference in this world. Inspire within me discipline to pursue Your truth and to cling to my confidence in You on a daily basis. In the saving name of Jesus, Amen.

30 DETOXES REVIEW GUIDE

1. Know that you only need to be you.

You are unique and were purposefully created by God. There is only one you, so stop wasting your time and emotional energy trying to be anything other than who you were created to be. All you need to do to honor God is to be the best version of who He created you to be.

2. Know that God has freed you from your past.

You are not defined by your past, but, rather, refined by it. You now have permission to let go of your past, to stop dwelling on it, and instead to use your energy to focus on maximizing life right now in the present. God has released you from who you used to be, He has forgiven you, and He has set you free.

3. Know that your thoughts can be trained.

The mind is the greatest tool we have available to us and we are fully responsible for how we use it. There is power in your thoughts—your thoughts have the ability to speak life or death over your potential and your purpose. By being intentional about your mental growth you can train your thoughts and control the way you think.

4. Know your thoughts have power.

Your thoughts determine the outcome of your life. Never underestimate the power of the words you think and the words you speak. By carefully crafting your thoughts, you can direct the destination of your life, your impact, and your influence. The thoughts you think give you the ability to enjoy life to the fullest.

5. Know that you are unique.

There is a reason why you are who you are, why you are how you are, why you look how you do, and why you were born where and when you were born. God has specifically created you for your life to tell a story and it is a story that matters. You have unique quirks, talents, interests, and gifts and they are all for a reason, so embrace them, embrace who you are, and trust that God will complete the good work He has begun in you.

6. Know that you are good enough.

Because it is God who created you, you are perfectly equipped to be who you were created to be. Furthermore, just by being you, you are enough. You are good enough. You have great worth. You have great potential. You have great purpose. You can stop questioning your value and start living with confidence because the pressure is off, all you need to do is be the best version of yourself you can be.

7. Know that you are loved.

God loves you because you are His child. There is nothing in the world you can do to earn more of God's love, and there is nothing you can do to lose His love. He loves you. Period. You have permission to stop trying to be perfect, to be impressive, or to reach a certain level of success in order to be lovable. You are loved because you are who you are. God is love. Trust in that, the most foundational and core identity of who God is. God loves you because He is love and because you are His child.

8. Know that you have greatness within you.

One of the most beautiful things about who God created you to be is that He created you to be special. You are different from anyone else and because of that, you have something great within you to offer the world. God created you to give something to others, to make a difference with your life that no one else can in the same way. Trust this greatness that God has breathed into you and develop it by trusting confidently in the person God created you to be.

9. Know that God makes all things possible in your life.

God can do anything. He is limitless and can perform miracles beyond human comprehension. Your mind is limited and has put limits on your life and potential because of self-doubt and fear. You can now live in God's omnipotent ability to do anything. With God by your side you are limitless.

10. Know that God has breathed into you potential and purpose.

You are here on earth because you have a purpose. It is a God-given purpose, and God has gifted you with the potential to fulfill it if you continue to walk in faith and in confidence, seeking to become the best version of yourself possible.

11. Know that you are remarkable and special.

There is something you have been given and have to offer the world that absolutely no one else has been given. You are special and have been specifically gifted accordingly. There is a reason why you live where you do, why the people who are in your life are in your life, and why you love what you do. Trust in who God created you to be and walk in confidence that He will put your gifts to good use so that your life leaves a real mark on the world.

12. Know that solitude is a way to grow in confidence.

One reason many people lack confidence is because they are too busy to notice and know what they can be confident about in themselves. Slow down the pace of your life; take time to get to know yourself, to understand your heart and to connect to the community around you by spending time by yourself. As you spend time alone you will learn more about who you are and about who God is, and you will be able to use this knowledge to walk more confidently when life gets noisy.

13. Know that life is about progress, not perfection.

One of the most beautiful gifts God has given us is that He doesn't expect perfection from us. He has given us perfection through the blood of Jesus Christ, His Son, and since that blanket of perfection covers us, all God expects of us is to walk the journey of our lives focused on the process of making progress.

14. Know that God is the ultimate Validator in your life.

You have a God-sized hole in your heart that longs to be filled. You cannot experience true happiness and full life until this hole is filled and it is only God's love that can fill it. When you allow God to fill your heart you will feel complete, validated, and fulfilled, allowing you to walk confidently in all that you do in life.

15. Know that real life happens when you walk your own path.

You have a path to walk, a race to run, that is your own. Real life, the abundant life that God has promised us, happens when we become trailblazers of our own journeys, walking out the story that God has written for us. You cannot live fully if you are distracted by comparing your race to anyone else's race; stay in your own race lane, walk your own path, and go live confidently the dream that God has put on your heart.

16. Know that you can choose the right perspective in life.

The way in which you experience the world is determined by the way in which you see the world. You have full control over your perspective and over the way you interpret your experiences in life. Choose the right perspective and you will see things in the world and in your life that you never imagined possible—with the right eyes, you can see God working actively in the day-to-day moments of life.

17. Know that God sees you as perfect.

You can let go of perfectionism because in God's eyes you are already perfect. There is nothing about you that needs to change or become better because God loves you as you are. That being said, there are certainly areas of your life and of yourself where you can experience growth and maturity, but the pursuit of those things has nothing to do with perfection or with you being perfect. There was only one perfect human being in the history of the world and that was Jesus Christ.

18. Know that you don't have to strive for perfection; you just have to strive to be yourself.

As you let go of the pursuit of perfectionism, you can now use that emotional and mental energy to invest in yourself in a more effective way. Rather than striving to be perfect, you simply only need to strive to be an authentic version of yourself. Strive to be who God created you to be and not an imitation of anyone else.

19. Know that you can fight fear by surrounding yourself with love.

The opposite of fear is love and you can fight any kind of fear in your life by saturating your mind with the truth of God's love for you. Fear cannot exist where love is, and where there is love, there, too, is God. Since God is everywhere and since He is always with you, you then have absolutely nothing to fear.

20. Know that you are allergic to negativity.

Negativity is toxic to your soul, your spirit, and your experience of life. Know that God created you to be allergic to negativity and avoid it with all of your might. Negativity is grounded in fearful, critical, and limited emotions and is not of God. By detoxifying negativity from your life you are making more room for positivity, for things of God, and for the confidence He can bring into your life.

21. Know that you are who you are meant to be.

You are one of a kind. Stop wasting time and energy trying to be like anyone else and instead use that energy to invest in your own personal growth and development so that you can be the best version of you that you can be. God does not make mistakes and He did not make any mistakes when making you.

22. Know that you have permission to dream big and do big things.

You cannot out-dream God or the plans He has for you. God has gifted you with potential and, if you choose to act on that potential, He will help you maximize it. The seed of greatness He has planted in you gives you all the permission you need to dream big and do big things through love in your life.

23. Know that God has your best interest at heart and that He works all things for your good.

The most important thing you need to know and believe about God is that He is good and that He loves you unconditionally. His love is the greatest thing that exists, and it is yours. And, since He loves us with such abandon and sincerity, He truly does have our best interest at heart and works out all things for our good.

24. Know that you are enough.

You have been created specifically by God and because of that you are a child of God, a child of *the* King. There is nothing that you can do to earn more of God's love and there is nothing you can do to lose it. You, as you are right now today, are enough.

25. Know that life is beautiful and God wants you to live it to the fullest.

Jesus came to earth and gave Himself on the cross to give the rest of us life, and life to the fullest. God calls this type of living abundant living, and He has made it available to us through His Son Jesus Christ. The invitation to abundant life is open, accept it and start really living life as it was intended to be.

26. Know that you have a legacy to leave and your story matters.

You can be a hero to this world, not by the big things you do, but instead through the small, daily, and consistent acts of love and kindness that you give by living your life with a heart of love. The legacy you leave to this world—and ultimately the impact you make—is a by-product of how you live in the small things. Your days matter, your story matters.

27. Know that confidence is available to you.

Confidence is a choice. It is a mental muscle and a conscious decision you engage with your own volition. You have all the confidence you need available to you through accepting and believing the knowledge that God has made you to be exactly who you are meant to be. You can be confident because God is with you in everything and with God there is only love.

28. Know that God's love is the foundation of your confidence.

Frame yourself and your life in the structure of God's love and by doing so you will always be grounded in confidence. You don't have to be confident on your own—that wouldn't be enough. Instead, you can be confident in the One who made

you His own, Who protects you and Who loves you unconditionally.

29. Know that the waves of your life have created great beauty in your story.

You are like beautiful sea glass that has been strengthened,
softened, and beautified by the rocking and rolling of the waves
of life. God has taken every trial and storm in your life, carried
you through it, and created in you more beauty because of it.
Even more exciting is that as life continues, and the waves
batter us even more, the beauty of our story will only become
more beautiful.

30. Know that confidence is something you renew daily.

Renewing your confidence is like flossing your teeth; to prevent mental plaque and negative buildup that could otherwise
be unnoticed, you must mentally floss your thoughts every day.

ACKNOWLEDGMENTS

This book would not have been possible without my hand-some husband Brandon Synan. Part editor, part coach, and full-time support team, his love and confidence in me has taught me more about myself and about God's goodness than I can possibly express. Thank you also to my parents, Diane and George Blackwell, who taught me that I can do anything I set my mind to, and to my brother, Nick Blackwell, who taught me how to explore the world and to trust my heart. I am who I am today because of the influence of a multitude of mentors and friends who God has graciously brought into my life . . . these people make me so overwhelmed with gratitude that my heart overflows. Specifically, I am grateful to the strong women in my life who have taught me what it means to have *joie de vivre* and how beautiful it is to be oneself—Kim Dickhut, Sharon Roberton, Nicole Sullivan, and Rachael Bodie. I owe my mentor and friend Todd Durkin a great expression of thanks for reigniting my courage and reminding me that I have a legacy to leave in this world that matters. I am eternally thankful for my amazing friends, Melissa Marquez, Angi Purinton Mc-Clure, Moe Nunez, Ved Miletic, Meghan Fillnow, Kelly Fillnow, Amanda Guerrieri, and Erin Guerrieri, who each in their own way give me the freedom to be myself and who celebrate beautiful living with me. Thank you to my agent, Ruth Samsel, for believing in me, believing in this project, and coaching me confidently through the process of this writing journey—here's to many more books to come! Thank you to Philis Boulting-house and all of the incredible folks at Howard Books/Simon & Schuster for having confidence in me and for making this book a beautiful reality. This book would also not be what it is without the magical editorial work and assistance of Nicci Jordan Hubert, who really helped my voice and stories come alive on these pages. I would also like to thank the amazing Christian leaders who are raising a generation in God's love and who have, without knowing it, spoken words of life, encouragement, faith, hope, and confidence into my spirit—thank you, Elevation Worship, Lifepoint Worship, Steven Furtik, Daniel Floyd, Craig Groeschel, Lysa TerKeurst, Patsy Clairmont, and Christine Caine. Most importantly, thank You, Jesus, for holding my hand through every moment of this beautiful journey of life.